Waiting for a Voice WITHDRAWN

The Parent's Guide to Coping with Verbal Dyspraxia

by

Sam Walker

Emerald Guide

British Library Cataloguing in Publication Data. A catalogue record for this book is available from the British Library.

ISBN

978-1-84716-482-7

Information in the nutrition chapter kindly provided by Katharine Tate.

Printed by Grosvenor Press London

Cover design by Bookworks Islington

This book reflects the ideas and opinions of the author, with the purpose of highlighting information on the topics covered in the book. It is not meant to provide health or medical evaluation, consultation or advice, and the reader is advised to consult appropriate health, nutritional and medical professionals for these services. The author and publisher therefore take no responsibility for any personal risk or loss.

This book is dedicated to the following people:

To Sue, a brilliant speech and language therapist, for being by our family's side every step of the way, and for helping Monty to find his voice.

To Katharine, my good friend, excellent nutritionist, and fish-oil provider. Thank you for everything, including the chickpea pasta.

Contents

****

Foreword

Working with Monty has been an amazing journey, which has involved many giant leaps forward and some small steps back along the way. His family have moved mountains to identify and implement a whole host of interventions that are collectively impacting on Monty's development. Sharing their experiences, understanding and awareness with other parents may prove hugely effective at making a real difference for so many others in similar situations.

This book is an honest, easy-to-read guide for those who are coping with verbal dyspraxia, including an up-to-date understanding of the disorder and identification of support strategies. Sam is a parent who is dealing with the disorder day-by-day and is working with a range of healthcare professionals and teachers to ensure all interventions that are deemed suitable are in place. This is a must-read for all parents who are also 'Waiting for a Voice'.

Katharine Tate

Nutritionist and Owner of The Food Teacher

(BEd (Hons), FAETC, Dip ION (Distinction), BANT, CNHC)

Katharine Tate is a qualified teacher, nutritional therapist, mum, and entrepreneur who has over 20 years' experience working with children in both primary and secondary schools in the UK, New Zealand, and Hong Kong. She has founded The Food Teacher brand to combine her passion for education and nutrition to deliver a healthy childhood, focusing on promoting family health through food and lifestyle.

INTRODUCTION
Imagine this, if you will.

About eighteen months ago I found myself sitting in an NHS speech therapy clinic room. It was a baking hot August day outside, there was only one window partially open in the room and everyone was fanning themselves with paper to create some breeze. My son, Monty, had just turned three and was there because he wasn't talking, and after various battles in actually getting him seen at the clinic, here we finally were. There were two Speech and Language Therapists (SaLTs) in the room, one asking Monty to do things ('Give the crocodile some dinner, Monty - does he want sausages or pizza?'), and the other therapist helping him to do as he was being asked. They were both nice and smiley, and Monty was quite happy and relaxed; there were lots of new and interesting toys to play with, and he did his best at imitating the animal noises that they wanted him to do ('Can you say *ahhhh*, Monty? What does the crocodile say when he opens his mouth?') I, on the other hand, was a bundle of nerves - there's nothing like wanting your child to 'perform' as expected when faced with a room of professionals and scribbling pens writing on clipboards.

Even though my husband and I knew that things weren't quite right with Monty's speech - we already had an older son and were therefore aware of the general milestones and what might be deemed to be 'normal' speech production in children - we still wanted someone to put our minds at ease and to tell us that there was nothing to worry about. I'd taken Monty to the doctors twice in the previous six months, and both times was told that he was a) a boy, and boys were often later to talk than girls, b), that he had an older sibling which had a tendency to make younger siblings late talkers due to having another small person to communicate their needs for them, and c), that the doctor's own son had been a late talker and hadn't spoken his first words until three years old. It also didn't help that Monty had made an attempt to say the word 'spider', completely randomly, in front of her on the second visit. Look – he's said a word! Nothing wrong with him, then! Case closed, and so out the door we went.

A self-referral a few months later to the health visitor resulted in a hearing test at the Audiology clinic, which showed that Monty had excellent hearing and therefore ruled out any hearing problems or ear complications like glue ear. The Audiologist, however, noted that Monty's speech was not very clear - I think she was being polite - and from then on, after several months on a waiting list, we found ourselves in this hot and stuffy room in the Speech and Language Unit.

After about forty-five minutes, and after many pages of notes had been taken, the lead therapist turned to me and said that it was clear that Monty had a speech disorder, most probably something called Developmental verbal dyspraxia. She asked if I'd ever heard of it - I said I hadn't. She then asked if I had any questions. Many thoughts were racing through my mind - the whats, the whys, but I went with a hopeful, 'I see. But - it'll resolve itself, right? Over time?'

I'll never forget the look of surprise on her face, as if I'd said something she'd not heard before. 'I'm afraid not,' she replied. 'It won't fix itself - Monty won't be able to talk clearly without intensive speech therapy, probably for a number of years.'

And then she added, apologetically, 'And I must warn you, there is at least a six month waiting list for speech therapy on the NHS in this area.'

We left the clinic and emerged into the bright sunlight; Monty walking along happily oblivious with his bag of toy dinosaurs, me clutching a handful of leaflets on speech disorders including 'Speech Techniques to Try at Home' and feeling like the bottom had dropped out of my world. I didn't cry until we'd got into the car, when Monty was safely in the back, munching on rice cakes, and then the tears fell silently into my lap as we drove home. I called my husband, and I called my dad. No-one quite knew what to say, although my husband vowed that we'd get it sorted.

That night, and for several days after, I cried quite a bit. I suppose it was the shock, that there was something 'wrong' with our precious little boy that needed 'fixing'. We told family members and a few close friends. I cried even more after getting the laptop out and Googling 'verbal dyspraxia' along with the words 'prognosis,' 'causes' and 'cures'. Apart from not being able to easily find out much about the condition, it concerned me how little the professionals actually seemed to know about it and how little research had been done in this country. Things became a little clearer after expanding my search to the USA, where there was suddenly a wealth of information available on the web, for the most part by parents that had set up their own websites or blogs to help others.

I started this introduction by saying, 'Imagine this.' Perhaps you didn't need to imagine this story, perhaps you have one somewhat identical or maybe similar to ours. Maybe you too have felt that there is a lack of information on the condition, like I did all those months ago. When I decided to write this book I wanted it, ultimately, to be the resource that I needed (and couldn't really find) when we, as a family, first set out on this long road of discovery.

This book is generally UK-based in terms of the terminology, and information on the education system and healthcare provision, but I hope it will also be useful for those reading in other countries.

13

I've tried to include much of the research I've done to date, and have provided where possible information on where you can find further help. As much as possible, I've tried to break it down into bite-sized chinks, which are hopefully easy to digest, and in non-medical language. In each section you will see boxes entitled 'A Parent's Perspective.' I felt that it was important to tell as much as possible about our own story, as this is a book not just about this particular life-changing condition, but the impact it has on the child, the parents and others involved in the family's life. Hopefully I may touch on some of the issues you may be experiencing, or may experience in the future, and with any luck can provide some sense of comfort that you will most likely not be alone in what you are going through.

I should mention here that I am not a speech and language therapist, nor do I have any speech and/or language qualifications (if you exclude the BA Hons degree in English Language and Literature!) I am an author, but I am foremost a mum, and this is the story of my family and how we have aimed to deal with verbal dyspraxia, which includes the things that have worked for us, the problems we have faced, and the research that I have done. What works for one child might not work for another, so always make sure that you consult a relevant professional before you try to implement anything new. I hope it points you in the right direction for finding the resources available, so that you can do your own reading and make your own informed decisions about what is right for you and your family.

The last thing to say, perhaps, is that you are not alone, and I and countless others have felt your pain. If you are just starting down this long and bumpy road, you are perhaps likely to find yourself becoming your child's advocate, speech therapist, stress reliever and taxi driver all rolled into one, in addition to the demands already found in a typical parenting role. Monty is only four, and I know we have a long way to go, but I also know we are doing everything we can to give him what he needs, to get him where he needs to eventually be, and you will no doubt be the same. In my heart, I know that we will get there.

I wish you and your child(ren) the very best.

Sam Walker

December 2014

Chapter 1

What is Verbal Dyspraxia?

___

Verbal dyspraxia. Developmental verbal dyspraxia. Articulatory dyspraxia. Apraxia. Childhood apraxia of speech. What do all of these disorders have in common?

Well the answer is... they are all the same thing. Confusing, right? Why not have just one name for a condition?

It seems there is no clear answer on that one, although it may stem from the lack of standardization in the past on the actual classification of the symptoms and the potential causes of the condition. The first three terms are usually the labels used within the UK, with the latter two those mostly used within the USA. In this book, for ease of use, I shall mostly refer to the condition as verbal dyspraxia.

So what exactly *is* verbal dyspraxia?

Verbal dyspraxia is a motor speech sound system disorder, which means that children with this type of speech disorder have difficulty making and co-ordinating the precise movements of the mouth, lips and jaw to enable clear speech production. 'Praxis' means planned movement, and therefore 'a-praxia' or 'dys-praxia' means a lack or absence of planned movement. It is a neurological condition, which means that it is linked to the brain and the programmed messages that the brain sends to other parts of the body - in this case, the mouth. It is not a language or developmental delay, which means that it is not that a child is following a typical route of language development but at a slower pace, or that children with verbal dyspraxia are 'behind' with their language and just need to 'catch up' - rather it means that the child knows what they want to say, but the messages from the brain to the oral structures of the mouth sometimes get scrambled for (as yet) mostly unknown reasons. It is common for a child with verbal dyspraxia to have typical receptive language abilities (understanding of language) whilst having severely affected expressive language (the ability to speak clearly).

In very simple terms, the child may want to say a word, of which the brain then passes on the message to the mouth and associated muscles, but something happens to make that message go awry, and the wrong movements are made and therefore the wrong sound comes out. I see it as being a bit like a motorway, where cars are busy going from A to B. Sometimes, cars don't receive the correct instruction from the sat nav, perhaps due to an unclear signal or the wrong information was input into the machine, and that can cause the vehicles to veer off onto a different route, which stops them from reaching the correct destination. If you apply that to the signals sent from the brain to the mouth, it means that in children with verbal dyspraxia the mouth and the neurological pathways do not connect in some way, and the mouth thereby receives the wrong 'message'. Perhaps it doesn't happen every time, and that is why some children with generally unclear speech can sometimes say a word quite clearly and correctly, and then appear to 'lose' that word for a certain amount of time.

Children with verbal dyspraxia have difficulty in producing the sounds required in speech, along with trouble in blending the required sounds to make words. Often there is also a difficulty with sequencing those words to make sentences. Not all children with verbal dyspraxia have the same symptoms, however, as it is what is known as a 'multi-faceted' condition and can present in children with different degrees of severity. At a basic level, the incorrect

18

patterns are stored in the brain, and therapy helps to re-train the teeth, lips and tongue and breathing mechanism to make the correct movements and shapes, and this new pattern is then hopefully stored as the correct method for future use.

Some children may also have, instead of or in addition to the speech sound system disorder, another condition occurring at the same time called Oro-motor (oral) dyspraxia, which affects the movements of the larynx, palate, lips and tongue, and may further inhibit the ability to produce clear speech.

Is it a common condition?

In some ways, yes *and* no. There are no clear statistics on how many people in the UK have 'pure' verbal dyspraxia (i.e. 'just' verbal dyspraxia and no other co-existing conditions.) The Afasic website in the UK state in one of their information sheets that 'most people typically assume SLI [specific language impairment] must be very rare, and are surprised that it affects nearly 7% of children (Tomblin et al, 1997).'[1]

The American Apraxia Kids website (CASANA) states that, of a typical speech and language therapist's (SaLT) caseload, probably only between 3-5% of those children with speech disorders seen have actual verbal dyspraxia, although that may be higher in relation to a specialist SaLT's caseload. It does appear that cases over the past few decades are more frequent, with more cases recorded, although this may be attributed to the narrowed, and commonly agreed, characteristics required for accurate diagnosis, earlier identification methods, and increased awareness by health

---

[1] Dorothy Bishop, *SLI: the invisible neuro-developmental disorder*, retrieved November 2014 from www.afasic.org.uk (download 303)

professionals. What is clear is that much more research and correct data collection is definitely needed. Verbal dyspraxia is, by nature, a changing, multi-faceted condition - indeed, some children find the label of their condition changing over time as new characteristics or difficulties present themselves. Also, it is known that having verbal dyspraxia may lead to other conditions presenting in the future, such as the development of an expressive language delay. All of this makes for a very grey area in terms of correct numbers of cases.

How do I explain that my child has verbal dyspraxia to other people?

I have found, over the past year or so, that people sometimes just don't seem to *get* what we tell them about Monty's verbal dyspraxia. My husband and I normally say something along the lines of 'Monty has a speech disorder, which means that sometimes the neurological pathways from his brain don't pass the message on properly to the muscles in his mouth, and the words come out a bit scrambled.' Sometimes that can be sufficient, however I often add that that it is a motor planning disorder, and that Monty is not 'behind' or 'delayed' (perhaps because I am a protective mum and I like to get the correct message across!). I think it can be hard for onlookers to process exactly what Monty's difficulties are, and the limitations of his social skills in some situations.

Of course, I don't go around telling every shop assistant what we are up against, but if the woman in the supermarket is expecting him to say thank you for something that they've handed him, or to answer their friendly questions, and he won't speak or make eye contact, it is then useful to have a short sentence prepared which tells them that he has difficulty in answering them and he's not being rude or difficult.

However, I think there is a point when too much information is, well, *too much* information. I remember the first time I felt uncomfortable about talking about verbal dyspraxia in front of Monty. We had gone to a theme park, where you can apply for a 'fast-track' pass to help with queuing if your child has certain additional needs. I was telling the man behind the desk, probably in long-winded detail about Monty's verbal dyspraxia and the challenges it produced, when I suddenly became aware that Monty was looking shyly at his feet. Was he fed up of hearing me talk about it to people? Did he feel embarrassed and uncomfortable? I decided then that I would try to avoid making a 'big deal' out of it in earshot of Monty, and to have a short sentence ready to quickly explain things without the lengthy detail.

If we're talking to children about Monty's condition, we tend to say that Monty is 'finding his words' and that his brain is working very hard to help him learn how to speak, and that we're sure he'll get there very soon. Children don't need to know the detail (not only will they switch off after the first sentence, it is also likely that the more you say, the more confused they may become.) And, let's be honest, it is a confusing subject for anyone to get to grips with, let alone a child.

The following is the basis of an email that I recently sent to the parents of Monty's new class at school. You might find it helpful when looking to offer your own explanation of the condition to family, friends, or new people that you meet. I tried to focus more on the positives (i.e. what Monty *can* do, rather than what he can't), and the fact that to all intents and purposes he is just like his peers and doesn't really need any 'special' treatment. Keeping the message short and cheery isn't likely to cause any offence, and the feedback I had was really positive from the other parents, as they then felt prepared for any questions that came home from their own children about why one little boy in the playground didn't talk very clearly and seemed to have his own language.

Here it is:

> *Hello all, Sorry for the mass email but I just wanted to tell you a little bit about our son, Monty.*
>
> *You might already have seen him doing a little bit of sign language in the playground, or chattering away to his classmates. Monty has a condition called severe verbal dyspraxia, which in a nutshell means that his mouth is often unable to process the messages that it receives from the brain, which in turn often means that his speech is unclear. Nothing else is affected, such as his understanding or his intelligence.*
>
> *Monty has speech therapy and we really hope that his condition improves. He obviously finds communicating a struggle, and can take a little longer than others to engage his brain to 'find' his words.*
>
> *On a happy note, Monty is a very social little boy - he loves play dates and parties, and is very happy to be at school.*
>
> *I just thought it would be useful to give you a heads up, in case your little ones have any questions - let me know if I can answer any! (I'll try!)*
>
> *Best wishes, and thanks for reading!*
>
> *Sam*

Some common characteristics of verbal dyspraxia

Only a Speech and Language Therapist can accurately diagnose verbal dyspraxia in a child, as they have the expertise and training to identify to the key characteristics that differentiate it from other speech disorders (more on that later.) Due to the fact that the condition changes over time and also presents differently with each individual, and the fact that an accurate identification and classification is also dependent on the age of the child and their ability to undergo assessment, it is widely accepted that it is a **complex diagnosis**. Some of the common listed symptoms are as follows:

❖ Having a limited range of consonant and vowel sounds
❖ Experienced feeding problems as a baby
❖ Had drooling as a baby, and/or lack of babbling sounds (quiet baby)
❖ An inconsistency of speech (can sometimes say a word, and then seem to 'lose' it)
❖ Difficulty with sequencing sounds and words
❖ Missing out parts of words, or substituting them with other sounds
❖ Problems with tone, pitch, volume and rhythm of the voice
❖ Weak mouth muscle tone

Often, but not always, there is a family history of speech and language difficulties, and/or problems with reading, spelling and writing. Monty had all of the above list, apart from feeding problems or drooling as a baby, and there is no family history of difficulties with speech. At his first assessment by the Speech and Language Clinic, it was established that he had only three of the five vowel sounds, and only one or two consonants, and only a handful of words that could mostly only be understood by close family that knew Monty well. We also knew that Monty, either then or at some point later, also had the following:

❖ Quite a bit of grunting in the early months, until the age of about three

❖ An initial lack of understanding of the concept of syllables

❖ Very slow progress in speech therapy, to the point that we spent a lot of the first 6-9 months mostly teaching him the same three sounds

❖ At first, an inability to blow air in and out through his mouth. It had never occurred to us that he *couldn't* actually blow out the candles on his birthday cake; instead we just thought that he didn't like blowing out candles...

❖ He could sometimes repeat words that we had said to him that surprised us, that would have been deemed too difficult, yet then not be able to do the same a moment later

❖ He would suddenly say a word or two, completely out of the blue, and then not be able to say that word for a very long time. For example, when Monty was eighteen months old, he said 'shoe' and 'fish'. We thought those words were the beginning of his ability to speak (what relief at the time – and yet how little we knew!) and it was very exciting. However, he wasn't able to say those two words for nearly another two years after that.

❖ Expressive language delay

❖ Poor auditory processing

❖ Limited voluntary movement of the tongue. It was difficult for Monty to poke his tongue out, for example, or move it to the top of his mouth.

❖ Pulling his face into positions with his hands (such as a kissing shape of the lips) to try to coax the mouth into the right shape.

Monty's speech, at 3 years old, typically consisted of repetitive vowel sounds, including 'ah' or 'ah ah', 'eh' or 'eh eh', 'ee' and various grunting sounds at the level of a 6-12 month old child, as was suggested by his speech assessment reports.

How is a diagnosis made?

A diagnosis is made by a speech and language therapist after assessment. Diagnosis can be complicated by having a mixture of common characteristics that may be similar to other conditions (see below), also by the age of the child (children need to be attempting speech for them to be observed and assessed, and if a child is too young that can prevent an accurate assessment taking place), the current level of development of the child, and also the fact that verbal dyspraxia often changes as it progresses. Most children under the age of two years 'do not have the ability to understand specific directions for tasks that would be critical to making the diagnosis.[2]' It is common to receive a diagnosis along the lines of 'John has a significantly reduced speech sound system disorder along the lines of a profound childhood apraxia of speech,' or 'Maisie presents with severely delayed expressive language skills and a speech disorder characteristic of verbal dyspraxia.'

A delay or a disorder?

There is a difference between a speech and language **delay**, and a speech and language **disorder**. A 'delay' generally means that children are learning to talk 'normally', but at a slower rate than other children, and a disorder means that speech or language is developing in an unusual way that is different to the typical model,

---

[2] www.apraxia-kids.org/guides/family-start-guide, retrieved November 2014

i.e. the language is 'dis-ordered' and a child needs help to rectify this, to learn the correct speech patterns. Rather confusingly, some professionals may use the term 'delay' to describe any type of speech and language difficulty. I have found that when I have mentioned the word 'delay' in relation to Monty's verbal dyspraxia, it can lead people to think that he is just behind with his speaking, perhaps akin to the abilities of a child of a younger age, and that people can sometimes get the wrong idea about the true nature of his condition and think that he will just naturally 'catch up' with his peers. For this reason, I tend not to use the word delay.

When children are very young, it can be difficult to determine which of these terms will relate to the difficulty they have in producing language and clear speech, which is why some professionals may want to wait to see how the difficulty progresses, before making an early diagnosis.

Similar conditions

There are a number of other speech disorders that have characteristics linked to verbal dyspraxia which accounts as to why it can sometimes be difficult to diagnose initially. If other conditions occur at the same time (co-morbidity) such as Autism or Down's syndrome, then language problems may be absorbed into another diagnosis. This can be a problem if it means that the correct type of therapy specific to verbal dyspraxia is not administered to deal effectively with the speech issues.

❖ **Dysarthria**

This condition relates to a weakness or low muscle tone in the lips, tongue and jaw that affects the ability to speak. Speech is often unintelligible, slow or slurred, and the person may have problems with drooling as they are unable to control the muscles

26

around the mouth. It may happen due to changes in the brain either before or after birth, or as an acquired condition caused by a head injury, stroke or as a result of Parkinson's disease. According to the NHS Choices website, unlike verbal dyspraxia, it may not always be possible to reverse dysarthria with speech therapy, although this depends on the extent of the damage to the brain, and the severity and development of the condition underlying the dysarthria.

❖ Aphasia

Aphasia is 'an impairment of language, affecting the production or comprehension of speech and the ability to read or write.'[3] It is caused by damage to the parts of the brain that control the use of, and understanding of, language, and is normally caused by a stroke or head injury.

There are different types of aphasia, but common characteristics include using short, stumbling sentences, with words missing so that either some or all of the meaning is lost; forgetting words (such as the aphasia often seen in Alzheimer's disease), and in some cases, the person not knowing that their spoken language is unclear to those that they are speaking to.

❖ Expressive language delay/disorder

Our expressive language relates to how we speak, in terms of output, and involves understanding the right words to use, how to formulate them into a sentence, and how to give the sentence the correct meaning .The Afasic website (www.afarsic.org.uk) gives the following explanation: 'Receptive language means the ability to

---

[3] www.aphasia.org/content/aphasia-definitions, retrieved November 2014

understand or comprehend language heard or read. Expressive language means being able to put thoughts into words and sentences, in a way that makes sense and is grammatically accurate.[4]

An expressive language delay may be diagnosed if the normal expressive speech production is slow to be achieved, but the general ability is there in terms of how to use words correctly, and how to follow the normal pattern and sequence of speech. An expressive language disorder would suggest, however, that acquisition is not only slow, but different from normal speech, and that the pattern of development is uneven and atypical. Children with a disorder of this kind may use language out of context, or use words in the wrong places.

❖ **Selective mutism**

Selective mutism is where a person chooses when and when not to speak. They may speak 'normally' at home where they feel comfortable in their surroundings, but then refuse to say anything at school, for example, or when expected to talk to someone they don't know. It isn't confined just to those children with a speech disorder, but it can be more common in those children who are naturally conscious of their speech ability and perhaps more wary of speaking in certain situations, or to certain people. It is seen as a psychological issue, where the child is not necessarily shy per se, but may be anxious for whatever reason.

---

[4] www.afasic.org.uk/recognising-a-problem, retrieved November

2014

Monty had selective mutism for several months, and only when he was in speech therapy, either at home or in the clinic. It used to drive me mad - on travelling to the clinic he would happily be babbling away to me, even singing sometimes, and as soon as we set foot in the door of the clinic, he sat in silence for the whole time. If we popped out of the session to use the toilet, he would then talk to me in the bathroom, making a few sounds that the speech and language therapist (SaLT) had been trying in vain to coax out of him, but would then be silent again as we re-entered the room.

On more than one occasion I asked if the SaLT had heard us in the bathroom, just to prove that he *could* speak (cue funny looks from her!) In desperation, we decided to move Monty's sessions to take place *only* in his education establishment, where it would be less 'clinic-y', and suddenly the situation reversed itself (thank goodness). I think also having me out of the picture for a bit took the pressure off Monty, *as hard as that felt at the time*. Perhaps he could sense my frustration, or he didn't want so many people looking at him when he was trying to do what was asked of him – I'm not really sure. I know that both I and his private speech and language therapist felt that he was against having speech therapy in our home after a while, as he seemed to feel that home was 'his territory' and he would get very cross with us both.

I suppose, in hindsight, our house was his only escape from the outside world, where he could just be himself and play with his toys and his brother, and not worry about his speech, but I didn't think of that at the time. Sometimes, it seems, a little trial and error is needed, until you find a solution that fits.

❖ Stuttering (dysfluency)

Stuttering, stammering and dysfluency are all names for the same condition. The condition is more common in boys, and approximately five percent of all children will suffer with some difficulty with their fluency at some time during the development of their speech.[5] Characteristics are very varied and differ between people, however they often include the repetition of single sounds (g-g-g-g-go), repetition of certain words (and, and, and) and no sounds coming out at all, even though the mouth is in position and appears to be trying to say the word. Again, similar to several of the other speech conditions discussed, the reason for acquiring a stutter is unknown. Therapy is available, and can be quite effective for some sufferers.

❖ Phonological speech disorder

A phonological speech disorder is categorised by a child using the incorrect sounds and words in their speech, and generally not following the 'usual' developmental pattern of speech. Often they may substitute some sounds with others, by producing the required sound in a different part of the mouth (i.e.'s' becomes 't') or by omitting the beginning, middle or ending of words, particularly where multiple consonants are together. Hearing difficulties should be ruled out, in case the child has been unable to distinguish the sounds they hear and re-produce them (for example if they have had many ear infections in childhood).

As you can see, there are many different types of speech disorders which, whilst different in cause and presenting symptoms, actually sound quite similar in many ways. So now we know why a diagnosis of verbal dyspraxia can be quite difficult to diagnose in some children!

------

[5] www.afasic.org.uk, (glossary12), retrieved November 2014

A note on Dyspraxia (Developmental Co-ordination Disorder)

Body dyspraxia, known usually as just dyspraxia, is a developmental coordination disorder (DCD) within the body that impacts on fine and gross motor abilities. Like verbal dyspraxia, the condition results in difficulty in planning, organising and carrying out movement. Common problems include a lack of balance and co-ordination which impacts on many daily activities such as writing, riding a bike and general use of fine motor skills. Other difficulties might include problems with time management, social skills and emotional behaviour. As with verbal dyspraxia, there is no known cause for the condition (although it is suspected that there is a problem with the correct messages being transmitted from the brain to the body), the symptoms and severity can vary with the individual and they can change over time.

The Dyspraxia Foundation states on their website that 'Current research suggests that it is due to an immaturity of neurone development in the brain rather than to brain damage. People with dyspraxia have no clinical neurological abnormality to explain their condition.'[6]

So what causes verbal dyspraxia, exactly?

Essentially, the answer to this is that the medical world aren't entirely sure. The CASANA (Childhood Apraxia of Speech Association of North America) website states that there are three potential reasons:[7]

---

[6] www.dyspraxiafoundation.org.uk/about-dyspraxia, retrieved November 2014

[7] Www.apraxia-kids.org/guides/family-start-guide, retrieved November 2014

- **Neurological impairment** caused by infection, illness or injury, before, during or after birth. Includes strokes or other brain injury.
- **Complex Neurodevelopmental Disorders** which incorporate verbal dyspraxia as a characteristic of another condition such as autism.
- **A speech disorder of unknown origin.**

There are also some suggestions that babies may be exposed to certain toxins or experiences in the womb which can cause developmental issues, although it seems that much more research needs to be done to investigate this.

➤ **A Parent's Perspective**

Monty was born, at 40+2 weeks, by normal delivery. I hadn't felt him move for about 24 hours, so I popped along to the birthing unit at our intended hospital to get them to check me out. The staff noticed that the baby's heart rate was exceptionally fast, and after a few hours of monitoring they decided that I would need to have a caesarean section, as it was possible that the baby was in some distress. Unfortunately, a nurse had been by with a sandwich and suggested that, as I was stuck at hospital for a bit, I should probably eat something. The Consultant was a bit cross when he came back, and told me that I shouldn't have had food before the procedure, and that on further discussion they were now going to wait and monitor the baby.

I was induced later that day, with Monty's heart rate continuing to race one minute, and drop the next. After a few hours of labour, my waters broke and the midwife said that they contained a lot of old meconium (the first stool that a baby passes, preferably when out of the womb) and that this can signify that the baby had been in distress for some time. When Monty was born not long after, the cord was wrapped round his neck, but otherwise he seemed ok. He was quite alert, and willing to suckle.

A few hours later, I found myself on the ward with Monty sleeping next to me in his hospital cot. Everyone else on the ward appeared to be asleep, and the room was uncharacteristically quiet. I remember looking over at Monty, next to the window, and the moonlight was shining in, right on him. I was watching him, lost in the tiredness and elation of labour and the relief that he was okay after what had been a very worrying day, when I realised that there was something strange going on with his breathing. As I leaned over, I could see through his blanket that his chest was swollen, almost like a barrel, and in horror I realised that he was struggling to breathe at all. I pressed the alarm bell, and before I knew it, I, and three midwives, were running through the corridor to the lift to take him up to the Special Care Baby Unit (SCBU).

From this point on, Monty was put on oxygen and stayed in an incubator to regulate his breathing. He had suspected pneumonia, which was then diagnosed as acute meconium aspiration, which means that he had inhaled the stool he had passed in the womb, and this was now on his lungs, with no way of clearing it by medical intervention. It was a waiting game, and one which scared our family out of our minds. Monty spent four days in SCBU, with some of the most gentle and caring specialist doctors and nurses I have ever come across, and to which we are eternally grateful for their dedicated care. I wasn't able to hold him for two days, and he had very little breast milk, but somehow Monty managed to pull through it all.

I have one other child, an older son, who did not have any problems at birth, who has no speech and language difficulties and who has followed all the usual milestones of typical development. Did Monty's birth experience and early days following birth have some impact on his brain's development? Did he suffer from a lack of oxygen? Did his start in life, and the large amount of antibiotics that most likely saved his life at the time, cause him to develop verbal dyspraxia? *Who knows*. Over time, I've come to worry less about the 'ifs' and 'whats' and 'buts', and learnt to deal with what I can control, in the moment... but it does still make me think.

How do we learn to speak?
Speech relates to the words that you say, whereas spoken language refers to the content of what is said. At a basic level, to make speech sounds requires the brain to store a pattern or a programme which tells the lips, tongue, teeth and breath what they should be doing to produce that sound, time and time again. To most people, this comes naturally as we learn from early childhood. Speech comes from an idea, an intention to communicate, which requires a sequence of sounds (also known as *phonemes*) to make words, all in the correct order. After the brain has told the correct muscles what to do, the muscles are then required to make the necessary precise movements. And this is all done automatically, without us having to think about it. According to the CASANA website (www.apraxia-kids.org), when learning to speak children 'make word attempts and get feedback from people around them and from their own internal sensory systems regarding how "well" the words they produced matched the ones that they wanted to produce. Children use this information the next time they attempt the words and essentially were able to "learn from experience."'[8] These plans or 'word maps'

---

[8] www.apraxia-kids.org/guides/family-start-guide, retrieved November 2014

are then stored in the brain, ready to be used the next time they are needed. It seems that the problem for children with verbal dyspraxia is that these word maps are either not formed or stored correctly, or that they have difficulty accessing them. There may also be issues with the sensory feedback that a child receives, either via their own hearing (auditory) system, or through the feeling in the mouth of where the parts of the mouth are, in order to 'feel' and then replicate the movement.

Also, learning to speak doesn't just relate to being able to produce sounds and words. Johan Langfield, a Speech and Language Therapist writing on the website www.icommunicatetherapy.com writes that 'speech and language skills do not just evolve on their own. They are part of a bigger picture involving social interaction, play, observation, manipulating objects, listening and attending. All these factors are working together and often, without one, it is difficult to develop another.' It is also important that the child practices listening exercises in addition to speaking exercises, as it is necessary to focus on listening to how the sound *should* sound, as well as working on the mechanics needed to produce it.

Learning to speak also involves establishing how to use language. The language we use is made up of many areas, including:

- Morphology - the way in which word structures change (for example, walk, walking, walked)
- Grammar - the rules about combining words in phrases and sentences
- Semantics - the way meaning is derived in language
- Phonology - the sound system of the language (phonetic sounds)

Add a speech disorder in to the mix, and you can see how things can get a bit tricky.

Prognosis

You may have noticed the 'childhood' element already mentioned (indeed, one of the American terms for verbal dyspraxia is **childhood** apraxia of speech) - it is a childhood disorder which gives hope for the fact that it may be resolved within the childhood years of life – with the correct help. Generally, it is accepted that the condition will not get better without regular speech therapy. It is also important that a correct diagnosis is made on the actual type of speech disorder, so that the correct type and amount of therapy is provided. There is, unfortunately, no magic cure. It is most important to identify it early, and to start speech therapy as soon as possible, and to ensure that the family are as involved as possible, with regular practice undertaken at home and school. It does depend on the personality of the child, but going on personal experience, I think the younger a child starts to have speech therapy, the more they may come to accept it as a 'normal' part of this stage in their life.

I have spoken to several speech and language therapists who have had brilliant success stories with the children they have worked with, with many going into adulthood with no hint of seemingly ever had an issue with their speaking and language abilities, and some still able to talk well with just a hint of an issue, such as tiredness when talking for long periods, or tiredness itself causing their speech to slip a little.

The Afasic website suggests that research shows that the longer that speech, language and communication needs persist into the school years, the lower the likelihood of them being resolved completely, although this comes down to the type of speech delay/disorder. Interestingly, they state that what children throughout later life might continue to struggle with, though, are 'the more subtle aspects of language they will increasingly encounter as they move up through school and into adult life – things like figures of speech, abstract concepts and complex sentence structures.'[9]

These listed 'higher level' language skills that may be lacking underlie the ability to:

- Make inferences, draw conclusions and interpret evidence
- Argue a case, explain your reasoning and express opinions
- Use and understand irony, sarcasm and word play

So, there we have it. Quite a lot of information to take in, you might be thinking. I have, at times, felt quite overwhelmed by the uncertainties about the prognosis of Monty's condition. These days, I do try to just focus on the problems of today, because I think if you worry too much about the future and what is to come, then the whole problem can seem like too much to handle, and if you are always obsessing about what **might** happen, then you are likely to be less present and focused on the things you can do **today**. It seems that where verbal dyspraxia is the only condition presenting in a child, then there is a very good chance that the child will overcome the condition.

---

[9] *Outcomes for Children with SLCN* (Retrieved December 2014, http://www.afasic.org.uk/recognising-a-problem/outcomes-for-children-with-slcn/)

Chapter 2

From Diagnosis to Action

As I mentioned in the Introduction, the moment you hear that your child has verbal dyspraxia, a myriad of emotions are likely to set in. As a start, some of the emotions you might be feeling could include:

- Sadness - you might feel that there is something 'not right' with your child.
- Denial – is this really happening? Is it really that bad?
- Fear - that this is a 'problem', with no quick fix, or clear prognosis.
- Overwhelmed - at the information (or lack of) provided.
- Grief- for the childhood and possibly adulthood you feel your child might not have.
- Worry - about the costs of speech therapy, communication aids, etc.
- Concern - for your child's future. Will they have a decent education, and go on to have a successful career that they enjoy?
- Fear - that they might not make friends, be included in social activities, or may be bullied.
- Anger - perhaps you think, *why us*?
- Guilt - There may be some guilt in the back of your mind that you might somehow have caused it (but be sure - you haven't).
- Worry - at the length of time that the condition might take to resolve itself, and whether *you* have the ability to sort it out.

- Concern - about the impact it may have on your job, your sleep, your concentration, and your relationships.
- Fear - that your family, especially your child's siblings, may be adversely affected.

Those feelings listed above are just those that I have felt at one time or another (and to be honest, some of them are still playing on my mind even now.) I remember once waking up in the night, sitting bolt upright in bed, with one thought in my mind - 'What if Monty can never leave home? What if he needs to live with us forever?' Not that I dream of the day that my children will leave home for university or a job, but I think it had suddenly struck me that Monty might not follow the route through life that could be available to him, whatever path he might choose. I also remember bursting into tears one day on the sofa, with my husband looking at me in alarm. 'What's up?' he said. 'I've just had a thought - what if Monty never meets a partner?' I replied. 'What if he's lonely when he's older?' My husband did the usual thing, of shaking his head, comforting me and saying that it would all be alright in the end, and that Monty would grow up to be just like his peers. But these thoughts would often pop into my head unannounced, catching me off-guard, and causing me to stop whatever I was doing in some frozen state of panic. What if? *What if*?

I think that it is important to let yourself feel these fears and emotions, as it is a natural part of the initial shock of having a child diagnosed with such a condition. There can be much gained from working through these fears, and allowing yourself to experience them, rather than bottling them up and ignoring them. Talk to friends and family members that you know will listen, without judging or telling you what to do. If you feel you need to talk to someone outside of your family or friendship group, you could

40

always make an appointment with your doctor to see what counselling services are available, or join a local support group. We didn't have one purely for speech-related disorders in my area, but I joined an additional-needs help group and met many other parents with children with autism, Asperger's and ADHD (amongst other conditions). I found that even though the conditions our children had were different, the feelings, emotions and daily struggles were consistent amongst many of the other women I met (bizarrely there were no male attendees!). Each time we met we would go round the group, asking what was going in in each other's lives, and hearing about some of the struggles and heartache, yet also the success stories in terms of treatment, successful school applications, and personal 'triumphs over adversity'. It felt good to have a supportive environment in which to off-load a bit of steam and worry.

Take time to let the diagnosis sink in, as well as any written report that you receive after your child's assessment. I find it best to read our reports once, making any notes of words that I don't understand and need to query (or Google), and then go back and read it again a bit later on. It's amazing how much you can miss on the first go, especially if you are worried or feeling a bit stressed out. If you can, make sure you have a telephone number or email address that enables you to contact the speech and language therapist who wrote it (or other professional, in relation to other reports you may have received) so that you can contact them if there is anything you don't understand.

Also make sure that the necessary people who are involved with your child's care (such as their school) have a copy. When you are ready, take your time to share the information with family and friends – sometimes it might be helpful for them to read the report as well, rather than just hear your version of the information contained within it, especially if they have a tendency to think that there is nothing really 'wrong'.

It is also important to show your child that they are not the only one out there who is learning to speak at their age, to avoid them feeling isolated, or somehow 'different' from other children. One speech and language therapist we met made a point of telling Monty that she was also seeing two more four-year-old little boys that day, to help them with their sounds and words, which I thought was a nice touch. One thing I have learned over the last year and a half is that children with verbal dyspraxia can often be far more aware of their speech difficulties than you might at first think, and they can often be very good at hiding this! I've found that some of Monty's coping strategies include not making eye contact, clamping his mouth together, repeating the same word over and over, and if he has been asked a question, to pretend that he hasn't heard it.

Remember, your child is still the same lovely little child that they always were. You now just have a 'label' to give to the problems they have been experiencing, and now that you have a name for the condition, you can do your very best to find out all there is to know about it, to give your child what they need to succeed. Knowledge is key. Your child will need your help, your time, and your support, and as their parent, you need no further qualifications to be perfectly qualified for the job.

And so to research...
I have to admit, when I first started to research verbal dyspraxia on the internet, I was quite shocked at the lack of available information on the subject, certainly from the UK-based websites. There was a certain amount of information on dyspraxia in general, but typing in 'verbal dyspraxia', even on the NHS Choices website, I was drawing a blank.

It's certainly clear that there hasn't been nearly enough research on the potential causes, contributing factors, prognosis and treatment process of verbal dyspraxia in the past, (certainly in the UK) but this seems to slowly be on the up. One of the main sites that holds the bulk of research and articles on the subject are those belonging to the American Journal of Speech and Language Pathology. It's an American site and unfortunately, on my last look, accepted payment for its journals only in US dollars from a US bank, which is a shame.

Lucky, the CASANA website (www.apraxia-kids.org) hosts a good selection of the most up-to-date research and key reports. Two of the most important pieces of research that I've come across on the site include:

- ASHA (American Speech Language Hearing Association) Technical Report on Childhood Apraxia of Speech (2007, www.asha.org).You can find the full report (74 pages!) on the www.apraxia-kids.org website. This gives a good overview of the condition, current research, previous studies, and gives a good argument for the advantages relating to treating the disorder if more research was to be undertaken in the future.
- Edeal, DM and Gildersleeve-Neumann, CE - *The Importance of Production Frequency in Speech Therapy for Childhood Apraxia of Speech.* American Journal of Speech-Language Pathology. May 2011, Vol. 20, 95 – 110. One of the key points in this is the necessity for constant repetition of speech sounds in therapy, as practice makes perfect, and also to incorporate actual speech into therapy sessions rather than just sound work on its own, to ensure that children understand that verbal communication is about

blends, words and sentences, not just individual sounds in isolation.

Do have a look under the 'Research' section of www.apraxia-kids.org – there are some great excerpts of articles and journals that include the latest findings on verbal dyspraxia and a whole host of other bits of useful information. It's also worth a trip to the library, especially if you have a University/academic library near you that also covers this discipline (try searches including child development/language/semantics/childhood speech disorders as a start.)

I'll discuss diet and nutrition in more detail in **Chapter 8 - Diet and Nutrition**, however I'll mention here that in relation to nutrition and alternative theories, I also like to keep an eye on the following internet searches, in case of any new information or research:

- Verbal dyspraxia/apraxia and ketogenic diets (there are on-going clinical trials to see whether a high fat/low carbohydrate diet has any impact on neurological/neurobehavioural conditions)
- Verbal dyspraxia/apraxia and childhood infections
- Verbal dyspraxia/apraxia and autoimmune conditions
- Verbal dyspraxia/apraxia and GAPS diet (GAPS stands for Gut and Psychology Syndrome).

The latter is a very interesting concept which you can read about in the book entitled 'Gut and Psychology Syndrome' by Dr Natasha Campbell-McBride. Dr Campbell-McBride writes about the issues that can occur within the human body if there is an imbalance of the gut microbes (flora and fauna), and puts across theories that many conditions like autism and verbal dyspraxia originate as gut disorders. Briefly put, she feels that if you can heal the gut, and stop a potential 'leaky gut' from allowing toxins that should have been disposed of within the intestine to enter the bloodstream and clog the brain, then there can be numerous benefits to children living with those types of conditions. It's probably not for everyone, especially those who favour the more 'scientific' approach, but I find it all very interesting.

Key professionals involved in caring for your child
With a diagnosis comes the inclusion of many healthcare professionals in the life of you and your child. At any given different time, you are likely to find a combination of the following professionals having an input into the care of your child, some on a one-off basis, and some for the long-haul:

❖ **Doctor (GP)**
A visit to the doctor is likely to be your first point of call (apart from the health visitor who may then refer you to your family doctor in the first instance). The GP won't be able to diagnose verbal dyspraxia or other conditions, but they are obviously able to refer you on to the correct professional.

❖ **Health Visitor**
It seems to differ in different parts of the country, and even within the same county, but generally your child will be offered a check-up with the health visitor at around two years of age. It was on the advice of our health visitor that I made the first appointment with our doctor, and it was eventually the same health visitor who made a referral to the audiologist to have Monty's hearing checked.

I liked talking through my concerns with our health visitor, as she obviously saw a lot of children of the same age and was therefore in a good position to assess whether she thought Monty's developing speech, or lack of, was consistent with other children in the same age-range.

❖ Audiologist

The role of the Audiologist is to test your child's hearing, and therefore rule out any hearing loss as a reason for their language and communication problems. They undertake specialized auditory (hearing) and vestibular (balance) tests to see whether hearing is within the normal range, and if not, which frequency is affected and by how much, and can refer on to the Ear, Nose and Throat department for further tests if needed.

❖ Paediatrician

A paediatrician is a doctor that specialises in children and babies. You might come into contact with a paediatrician that specialises in audiovestibular medicine, a specialty relating to hearing and balance, alternatively you might see a community paediatrician. The Royal College of Paediatrics and Child Health website states that:

'Community Child Health is the care of children outside hospital. {...} Community paediatricians see children as outpatients for a variety of reasons and their patients can include children with long-term disability (e.g. cerebral palsy, learning disability), children with mental health issues (e.g. autism and ADHD), children who it is feared are being abused, or children who are being fostered and adopted. They also take responsibility for advising on the health of communities. Some community paediatricians work in the highly specialised area of audiology, looking after children with severe hearing loss.'[10]

Monty has seen both a community paediatrician and a specialist paediatrician in audiovestibular medicine, and it is clear that the specialisms do differ in what they are looking for. Both were keen to find out about Monty's history, and check his height, weight and body measurements. I think the community paediatrician was most concerned about his ability to cope and function in the school environment; any genetic contributing factors that might need ruling out (she raised some concerns that his slightly flat head could be a marker), and his long-term needs. The paediatrician specialising in audiovestibular issues was most concerned with looking at the working of Monty's mouth, his actual speech production and articulation, and whether any long-terms effects might result from his verbal dyspraxia (such as the condition later presenting as an expressive language disorder or delay.)

❖ **ENT (Ear, Nose and Throat specialist)**

Your child might be referred to the Ear, Nose and Throat department for further tests if it is suspected that any of these parts of your child's body have something to do with their speech difficulties. ENT doctors are called Otorhinolaryngologists (try saying that out loud!) and they look at tinnitus, vertigo, glue ear, ear infections, nasal obstructions and other conditions.

❖ **Speech and Language Therapist (SaLT)**

The person soon to become a major part of your life! A

---

[10] www.rcpch.ac.uk (paediatric sub-speciality glossary section, retrieved November 2014)

speech and language therapist will work with you and your child, normally in clinic or they may also visit your child's nursery or school. The Royal College of Speech and Language Therapists website states that SaLTs work with children with mild, moderate or severe learning difficulties, physical disabilities, language delay, specific language impairment, specific difficulties in producing sounds, hearing impairment, cleft palate, stammering, autism/social interaction difficulties, dyslexia, voice disorders, and selective mutism.[11]

The role of the SaLT is to assess the child's needs, providing a diagnosis where possible, devising and implementing a treatment plan, and to monitor their progress. They will liaise with the education provider, write reports to give guidance for inclusion in an IEP or Statement of Educational Needs/Education, Health and Care Plan, and give advice to other professionals involved in your child's care.

Please see **Chapter 3: What to Expect in Speech Therapy** for more information on the role of the SaLT, and the differences between NHS and private therapy.

❖ **Nuffield Centre for Verbal Dyspraxia**

The Nuffield Centre is based at the Royal National Ear, Nose and Throat Hospital (University College London Hospitals) in London. It is 'a multi-disciplinary specialist centre for the assessment, diagnosis and management of hearing disorders, listening difficulties, speech and language difficulties, tinnitus and balance disorders in children and young people from birth to 19

---

[11] www.rcslt.org/speech_and_language_therapy_what_is_an_slt (retrieved from website November 2014)

years of age.'[12] The current referral guidelines are as follows:

- The referral must come from a GP, Speech and Language Therapist or other associated healthcare professional
- The child must be three years old or more
- The child should have difficulty making speech, with frequent errors
- The child should have already have been receiving local speech therapy

Normally on arriving at the centre you will be seen by a doctor (paediatrician) and a speech and language therapist with much experience in verbal dyspraxia. Monty has been twice, and after the second visit we received a detailed report about his condition. The appointments can be quite long – Monty was assessed on his speech ability for nearly an hour on the second appointment and nearly feel asleep on my lap afterwards – so go prepared to be there for some time, especially if there is a delay and you are kept in the waiting room for a while. Sometimes the Centre may offer a short course of intensive therapy at a later date if they feel it will be of benefit to the child, often in the school holidays.

❖ **Occupational Therapist**

An occupational therapist can be helpful in showing an individual how to adapt the activities that they need to do, in order to make them more manageable. They can help with introducing

---

[12] www.ndp3.org/about-the-nuffield-centre (retrieved from website November 2014)

games and activities to practice that aim to improve social skills, concentration and movements of muscles in the body, and to advise on any equipment that might be useful to aid communication.

❖ Educational Psychologist

An educational psychologist may be involved where a child is, or may be, having difficulty in the education environment due to emotional, psychological or behavioural factors coming into play. I will talk further about the role of the Educational Psychologist's role in **Chapter 5: Education**.

➢ A Parent's Perspective

Even after all this time, it can be daunting having to meet yet another professional who needs to have an input into your child's care . It is tough having to explain yet again the complete history of your child's life, from your birthing story onwards to the present day. I often wonder if anyone reads other healthcare professional's notes, but I've come to see it that they are often looking for that missing link, and that hearing the story first-hand is important, in case a new line of questioning brings to light a golden nugget of information. I've got our story honed down to a tee now, as I know what information is necessary. Making notes is very useful, in case you feel you might miss something out at an appointment.

A word on 'playing ball' - and I don't mean in the sporty sense! Monty has become very self-aware in the clinic environment - he can spot a yellow-painted room with a table and chairs and building bricks a mile off these days, and he seems to know that he is there to be 'assessed' and observed, so he develops varying degrees of selective mutism; i.e. he chooses not to speak which can be very frustrating for all involved and often feels like a wasted visit.

If this happens with your child, do make sure that you discuss it with the professional involved. I was so worried that Monty was refusing to attend his speech therapy sessions, that we tried moving the room (not much change), we tried removing me from the sessions so that he might behave better (small improvement, but left me frustrated as I didn't know what was going on), and also introducing new and exciting toys into the session (a little bit better). Even having our private speech and language therapist come to the house made Monty run to the end of the garden and hide behind the trampoline.

Finally, I took the decision to stop his sessions being in the at home or in the clinic setting. And bingo! Suddenly Monty was ready to take part. We moved all sessions to his education environment (firstly nursery and then reception class at school) and I have to say, we have never looked back.

I think sometimes you need to keep trying things, until eventually something clicks and the cycle is broken. It might mean having a short break from therapy, changing therapists, or changing the way in which a service is delivered. In short, if things aren't working for you, don't be afraid to change them.

How to prepare for appointments

It is useful to think about and write down the following, so that you don't find you've missed things:

- Pregnancy history, for all children you have had
- Your birthing stories and any complications
- The early days after the birth of your child
- Medication history for you, your partner and your child
- Development of your child
- Allergies
- Family history of speech and language difficulties

- What made you seek help for your child in relation to their speech
- What your child likes and dislikes
- Social aspects of your child's life, and how they respond to different situations
- Dates of first babbles, sounds, words.
- List of sounds or words you have heard your child say to date.

What to ask before and during appointments

There have been countless times when I have left an appointment with a doctor, therapist or consultant, with my head spinning from all of the information given, only to kick myself when I've returned home realising that I never asked the right questions, or forgot to ask something really important. So I would suggest that before you attend an appointment, you think about the following:

1) What is the appointment about?

Read all correspondence carefully, and don't hesitate to ring the office number if you have any questions beforehand. Also, check that the address you think you are going to is actually the correct place! Some hospitals have the main site address at the top of the letter, but are actually arranging for you to attend a clinic that is not on the main site, which could even mean it is in a different town altogether.

2) Who will be there, what is their role, and should anyone else also be at the meeting?

I have been at meetings where nothing could be agreed because key professionals were not there, and therefore the lack of representation from their particular service held things up. It can also cause delays when people have to be brought up to speed, or diaries have to be aligned for another meeting. These professionals are generally busy people, and re-arranging appointments to suit all can, in my experience, cause much delay.

3) Is the presence of your child requested, and/or are they asking for no siblings to be present?

There may be some meetings that your child will need to attend, for example assessments, but others such as Statement of Educational Needs/Education, Health and Care Plan reviews do not usually require the attendance of your child, unless otherwise requested. Siblings can be a distraction, both to the child and adults in the room, and they can impact on your ability as a parent to concentrate and take in all that's being discussed.

4) Do we need to bring anything with us?

As a first, I would always take the confirmation letter with you, in case you forget who you are seeing and where you need to go. You might also need to take any previous reports or notes, your child's medical records, and possibly if you have a small child, their red book which contains birthing history, immunisation history, etc. A notebook and pen are usually necessary to make notes in, and your diary should you be asked about future availability for further appointments when you are there.

If your child is attending with you, I would also suggest that you take a bottle of water and some snacks, and some books or toys to alleviate boredom during the inevitable waiting-room stint. A change of clothes wouldn't go amiss, either - I once took Monty to see his paediatrician dressed in some pink girls' leggings, as he had a little accident with some ice-cream in the car on the way there (a little bribery to get him there!) and the only spare clothes in the car belonged to a friend's little girl. Thank goodness he was young enough not to really notice, let alone mind!

5) <u>What are the outcomes likely to be?</u>
Are there any referrals that this meeting needs to provide, to other departments (for example audiology, or the ENT?) When will we need to see you again?

During an appointment
During any meeting, you might also like to have the following questions in mind to ask, depending on where you are and who you are seeing:

1) What are the differences in the treatment/therapy/written plans that are available?
2) What are the pros and cons of what you are suggesting?
3) What are the likely outcomes, for example in prognosis, timescales, amount and frequency of therapy needed?
4) Have you much experience of this type of condition?
5) How severe is it?
6) What is the prognosis, and what could affect this from being realised in the future?
7) Can you suggest any alternatives in addition to what you have deemed necessary?
8) Are there likely to be any costs to us, as a family?
9) What research is currently being done in this area?
10) Are there any other departments/professionals that we might also benefit from seeing?

Treatment
This could probably have been the shortest section in the book! The

only way to treat verbal dyspraxia, in terms of giving your child the help they need in order to achieve clear speech, is for them to attend regular speech therapy.

Some different Speech and Language Therapy Programmes

- The Kaufman Speech to Language Protocol (Kaufman) (USA)

The Kaufman approach was developed by Nancy Kaufman (www.kidspeech.com) and aims to teach children with verbal dyspraxia and other speech-related conditions to learn to speak via word approximations (by learning the easiest way to say a word, and them working towards correcting and refining that word until it is correct). The website explains that '[Children] are actually taught the shell of words without including too many of the complex consonants, vowels, or syllables which make a word too difficult to even attempt on a motor basis.'[13]. The Kaufman materials include visual cards, treatment kits and workbooks to progress through.

- Speech-EZ (USA)

The Speech-EZ system is another popular programme in America.

The programme uses hand clues and gestures to help the child remember individual speech sounds, which then act as a visual prompt when the child is learning and then aiming to recall the correct plan for speech production. It states on the organisation's

---

13

www.kidspeech.com/index.php?option=com_content&view=article &id=71&Itemid=460 (Retrieved from website December 2014) website that, 'Gesturing helps speakers to organize spatial information for verbalization, playing a role in conceptualizing the verbal message. A child using gestures and symbolic hand cues during speech production has enhanced access to items in their mental representation of sounds and movement planning for speech. Movement helps movement.'[14]

Interestingly, the website reads that, in relation to speech therapy frequency, 'research has proven that shorter but more frequent sessions (30 minute sessions; 4-5 times a week) are more effective and more efficient than longer, less frequent sessions such as 60 minute sessions; 2 times a week).'[15]

- PROMPT (Prompts for Restructuring Oral Muscular Phonetic Targets) (USA and UK)

This programme looks to aid the development of motor skills to assist in the development of language, as a multi-dimensional approach that uses touch to guide the lips, jaw and tongue into the necessary positions to achieve correct speech (be that sounds, words or full sentences.)

Monty's private SaLT has used this in the earlier sessions we had, when it seemed that Monty didn't have a clue where to put his tongue or lips, and he was gently guided to feel where his tongue needed to go, or the shape his lips needed to be. He was also shown

---

[14] www.speech-ez.com/apraxia-clinic.html (Retrieved from website December 2014)

[15] www.speech-ez.com/apraxia-clinic.html (Retrieved from website December 2014)

where the vibrations or 'feeling' would be upon certain sound productions (such as when you make an 'n' sound, if you press the side of your nose you can feel it vibrate.) I found this very useful and something we could replicate at home, and it was also informative for me to experience it as well.

- NDP3 (UK)

One of the main speech programmes for children with verbal dyspraxia in the UK is the Nuffield Centre Dyspraxia programme NDP3. It is a motor skills programme, used widely throughout the UK, and one which Monty has used from the very start. The Nuffield Centre describes it as a 'bottom up' approach, in that the aim is to 'build accurate speech from core units of single speech sounds (phonemes) and simple syllables.'

The website also states that 'new motor programs for single phonemes and words of different levels of phonotactic structures are created and perfected using cues and feedback. They are established as stored representations by associating them with pictorial images and through frequent practice and repetitive sequencing exercises'.[16]

Monty has spent the last year or more working on individual sounds, starting with those that he had already mastered, and only moving on to new sounds once those that he'd been working on were established. Each week we get homework, with new sheets from the NDP3 programme to work on, with repetitive sounds 'oo, oo' and/or blending sounds (ah, mm - ah, mm- 'arm'.) The sheets consist of little pictures that each represent a sound (the crocodile

---

[16] www.ndp3.org (retrieved from website December 2014)

opening his mouth represents the sound 'ahhhh', for example.) Once a child is able to move onto actual words, there are then pictures which are representative of the object that they depict. It might sound confusing, but once you get started it does make sense. One of the most important things for you as a parent to do is to make sure that you know how the different sounds should actually be *said*, because if you are saying them wrong then that won't be helping your child. I remember confusing one of Monty's SaLTs last summer when I asked how the 'w' sound on the Nuffield programme should be articulated – we were doing more of a short 'phonic' sound at home 'w', whereas in clinic Monty was asked to do more of a 'wooo' sound (like a ghost).

I felt a little confused about how a programme like this would work at the beginning, but once I'd looked at the NDP3 website it became clearer. The programme is set out on a brick wall, which literally shows you the stepping stones (up the 'wall') that lead to clear speech production by establishing the motor programmes necessary for each level. The NDP3 website describes it as 'speech skills are conceptualised as a "brick wall", with pre-speech skills and single consonant and vowel sounds seen as the foundations, and word level skills built up in layers of bricks on top of the foundations.'[17]

These steps are as follows:

- Single sounds (a/ah/ee etc)
- CV words (consonant/vowel words, such as he)
- CVCV words (consonant/vowel/consonant/verb words, such as 'cake')

---

[17]   www.ndp3.org/dyspraxia-praxia-treatment-approach (retrieved from website December 2014)

- CVC words (consonant/vowel/consonant words, such as 'cat')
- Multisyllabic words
- Consonant cluster words
- Phrases and sentences
- Connected speech (the Holy Grail!)

Whilst we are on the subject, I think it is useful to consider what the 'normal' speech and language milestones are in children. In *Speaking of Apraxia – A Parents' Guide to Childhood Apraxia of Speech*, the author Leslie A. Lindsay gives a breakdown of some of the key elements of ability that are often realised in each specified age group. Whilst Leslie points out that no two children are the same, these comparisons are useful when you are trying to establish how your child might compare to others of the same age.

For example, Leslie writes that at age 2-3 years, a child is likely to understand about 900 words, be able to say about 500 words, and has speech that is understandable about half of the time. A child of age 3-4 years is likely to understand about 1200 words, use about 800 words, and be able to be understood about 70-80% of the time.[18] Interestingly, other milestone breakdowns can differ slightly in opinion – if this subject is something that you are keen to explore, you can research on the internet using the terms 'child development speech and language milestones,' via some of the organisations already listed, or via those listed in Chapter 10 – Further Reading.

The brilliant American website, www.apraxia-kids.org, has

---

[18] Speaking of Apraxia – A Parents' Guide to Childhood Apraxia of Speech (Woodbine, 2012) p.419-420

some fantastic help sheets that give guidance on the types of therapy and the way in which therapy is given to an individual child, depending on their needs and abilities.

The following contains an adaptation of the list written by Sue Caspari in the help sheet, Treatment Approaches for Children with Childhood Apraxia of Speech (CAS)[19]:

- ❖ *Multi-sensory cueing techniques use sensory cues to help the child hear, see, feel, and understand the target speech movement gestures being requested of them as they practice words or phrases.*

- ❖ *Integral stimulation approaches use a well-defined and structured hierarchy of speech targets and require the child to imitate utterances (syllables, words, or phrases) modelled by the therapist. In this approach, the child's auditory attention is focused on listening to the words, and his visual attention is focused on looking at the therapist's face. Over time as the child's skills improve, the therapist varies the timing of the child's repetition and then works toward the child's self-initiated correct production of speech targets.*

- ❖ *Progressive approximation and shaping techniques use speech productions that children are currently capable of producing and then, through various forms of feedback and practice, attempt to shape the child's movement gestures into closer and closer approximations of the target word.*

- ❖ *Phonetic placement techniques provide verbal information*

---

[19] Sue Caspari, *Treatment Approaches for Children with Childhood Apraxia of Speech (CAS)* BSHM Factsheet 2, (retrieved from www.apraxia-kids.org December 2014)

and instruction to the child regarding what to physically do with their mouth, tongue, lips, or jaw during speech attempts in order to achieve more accurate articulatory positions for certain sounds that may be difficult for them to produce. However, the main focus of speech therapy is on speech movement sequences.

❖ ***Tactile facilitation approaches** use touch or manipulation of the head, face, lips and jaw during speech production so that the child can better "feel" and over time remember how to move their articulators correctly in order to produce the speech movements. Assistance is often provided at first and then faded as the child obtains independence at making the movements gestures for speech.*

❖ ***Prosodic facilitation** uses rhythm and melody to provide timing or rhythmic structure within which speech movements can be achieved.*

Action plans relating to Speech and Language Therapy

Ideally, after a speech and language assessment, you will have been given an overall plan for what needs to be achieved and where your child is heading (perhaps as a monthly plan, or as a three to six month target). In Monty's case, we have also been fortunate to receive weekly write-ups which lists targets for the session; outcomes that happened within the session (what occurred, what went well and what needed more work, and the level of difficulty experienced); things to continue at home; recommendations for activities; observations or key points, and the plan for the next forthcoming session(s).

I've been reviewing all of our weekly sheets since our very first session, which I share with you below in the following boxes. The reason for doing so is to firstly show how things can be slow-going for much of the time, and you may find that you are spending many weeks or months on the same types of exercises, or the same sounds and words until they become ingrained and the speech patterns and plans are learned and easily recalled. Secondly, and with a big *whoop-whoop*, I want to show how sometimes, you can have what can only be seen as some sort of breakthrough, whereby something, *somehow*, seems to be clicking into place. One of our first action plans of things to continue with at home from September 2013 looked like a longer version of this (below.) At the time Monty did not have any clear words, and had only three vowel sounds and one or two consonants.

Sept 2013

- Continue with soft blowing (use tissue, cotton wool) and hard blowing (party blower, whistle, etc.) to help with lip movements to realise 'p', 'b' 'm' sounds. Use straws to blow out (try table football), and to drink liquid.
- Try VC words with pause ('arm' – 'ah/mmm')
- Work on vowel sounds – 'ah', 'ee', 'I'.

Things pretty much continued at the same pace for nearly a year, with a few short bursts of progress, a small backwards step in which Monty seemed to 'lose' the words he did have, and a general difficulty in being able to do the blowing and breath control that was required. He would tire quickly, yet would have some pleasure in being able to make the whistle or other object make a sound/fly off the table, and would pull his lips into the shape needed with his hands. He seemed frequently to be unable to replicate facial movements that the SaLT and I would model for him.

The next action plan I've included is from one week's session from August 2014. As you can see, some of the sounds we were working on at this point were the same as in the previous action plan eleven months beforehand, but it also shows that Monty was successfully saying several words with great success – words such as Mummy, arm, fear, farm, ice, nice, house, hair, hat and mouse. Monty could also put two of these words together, such as 'Mummy arm', 'mouse house'. At this point, he couldn't say his name.

August 2014

- Continue with blowing techniques and tongue 'press-ups' to touch the roof of the mouth.
- Continue to practice vowel sounds ('ah', 'ee', 'oo', 'ow')
- Copy consonant sounds ('s', 'sh', 'f', 'h', 'm' already realised) (keep trying for 'l' and 'p')
- Continue to practice VC, CV, CVC words already working on
- N.B. Monty successfully realised 'sh', 'ow', 'er', 'f', 'ar', and 'm' sounds in the session today. (Shower, farm, in sections)

Within three to four months after August 2014, something seemed to click, and Monty took a greater interest in his speech therapy sessions. He started to ask me most mornings if he would be seeing his speech and language therapist that day, and he began to take great pride in his speech folder and would want to get it out of his book bag as soon as he got home from school, ready to continue where he had left off during the school day. How did this all come about? I put it down to a combination of things, including starting school, being in a focused learning environment, starting to learn phonics at school, and I think slowly accepting that doing the therapy was making a difference to his life. Monty's attitude to speech therapy (which changed from cautious interest, to denial, and then to outright refusal to participate over many months) was now in full-on co-operation mode (and what a relief!)

Our most recent plan for speech work at home looks like this:

December 2014

- Practice breaking words down into the correct number of syllables (for example, elephant would be three taps or claps – el/ee/phant)
- Sequencing of rhyming words (me, tea, pea, key for example)
- Work on a sentence a day, such as 'My name is Monty', 'I am four years old'.
- Build on making existing sentences longer
- Work on 'f' sound to ensure blowing out, not sucking air in

---

Look at how long we have spent on some things, and then how quickly things can move on, almost out of the blue. There are some new, exciting additions (Sentences! Who would have thought!) There are also some bits in there that keep us on our toes – Monty had really nailed the 'f' sound previously and could say it beautifully, but for some reason he had started to suck the air in when saying it, rather than forcing the air out. I wanted to share this with you, for the purpose of showing that it can be a long, frustrating process; it can seem that you are not progressing, and your child is not taking it all in. It can take some time, but then suddenly, things really can start to fly. Sometimes, it really is amazing how things can move on, even in a matter of weeks!

Alternative methods of communication

Whilst you will obviously be wanting to make sure that your child receives the necessary speech therapy in order to enable them to be able to speak, it is often a good idea to look at alternative methods of communication in the meantime to enable your child to feel that they can express themselves in a way that feels comfortable to them. Often, for a child with 'pure' verbal dyspraxia without any other co-occurring conditions, that is expected to eventually be able to use speech as the predominant form of communication, the ideal option is to use Makaton.

> ➤ **A Parent's Perspective**

When we realised that Monty's speech disorder was going nowhere fast, we knew that we had to do something to help him communicate his needs a bit better than by just grunting and pointing at things. It suddenly occurred to me that I wasn't helping him by giving him the things he wanted, for example a drink of water, by just handing it to him when he pointed to the cupboard with the glasses in it. If I wasn't there for some reason, how would anyone looking after Monty know what he was asking for?

Also at this point in time, Monty was having quite a few frustration tantrums each day, whereby his inability to communicate very clearly affected him. He was able to hold it in at nursery, but would 'unleash the beast' when safely back in the confines of our house. It wouldn't take much - perhaps I would just have had to ask him to repeat a word a couple of times because it really wasn't clear what he was asking for, or perhaps Monty would be trying to describe an activity he'd done that morning or a friend he'd played with, and I'd not been able to understand. You could see the frustration rise up in him, and he'd lash out, scream, stamp his feet or all of the above. It was worse though, for me, in the few

65

times when he would look defeated and just walk off. This worried me, because when I saw the shutters coming down, I felt that he'd seen it as an easier option to just give up trying, and this was far worse than him getting cross, in my opinion. At the same time, Monty had suddenly become very savvy about expecting us to repeat everything that he had attempted to say back clearly to him, in order to check that we weren't just agreeing with him to keep the peace! This was an exhausting time, and a period whereby as parents we felt we were forever walking on eggshells, afraid to put a foot (or word) wrong. Nursery had given a us a pack of laminated faces depicting a particular emotion stuck on lolly sticks - one for sad, one for happy, one for cross and one for confused/worried. Monty carried these around with him for a week or two, but he soon chose to stop using them, perhaps because there was only a small number of times when he felt they came in useful.

It was during one of our early speech therapy sessions that the subject of Makaton was brought up as a suggestion to give Monty assistance in making himself understood. Again there was a long waiting list, but after the speech and language therapist referred us on, both my husband and I managed to get on the course within a few months. We found it really useful - two mornings in total, and we came backed armed with the book of signs and symbols that had been very simple and quick to learn. With a bit of practice, and the book on hand in case one slipped our memory, Monty had soon learned the signs for family members' names, colours, animals, and activities in daily life such as washing, eating, and needing the toilet. A revelation! Suddenly there was a means of 'talking' within the family that we could all do (and learn) together, and I think it made an enormous difference to Monty's confidence and emotional well-being that he suddenly had another means of communication. It also probably helped that he could see we were all starting out from the same place - as beginners learning a new language.

Makaton

Makaton signs are taken from British Sign Language (see below). It is a basic, easy to learn sign language used from baby up to teens or beyond, encompassing the basic needs through to being a full communication system. You might have seen Mr Tumble in the television programme *Something Special* using Makaton signing. Each sign has a symbol to ensure that literacy skills can develop, and these can be used on visual timelines and time tables, to show the sequence of events and the order in which they are happening. For example, in a nursery or school setting the symbols for snack, play, group time, lunch-time are arranged in a linear form to show what is happening now, and what is coming up next. Communication boards and choice boards that also use symbols are a useful tool - the child can carry them around and use them to point to communicate a need, or to choose between items (such as food at snack time.)The symbols are also used to aid writing, teaching, and in the production of books and leaflets and other information. Have a look at the PECS system (Picture Exchange Communication System) – this has a systematic approach to building communication skills and developing sentence structure, as well as confidence. There are a variety of software programmes and apps that can be downloaded - we have My Choice Pad, which gives you some of the symbols for free, and the rest you can download for a fee.

The Makaton Charity, in addition to developing over 11,000 concepts in both symbol and sign form, offers training for tutors and workshops for parents and teachers, teaching resources, controls a list of licensed tutors available, and provides translation services. I went on the Beginners Workshop which was run by a local NHS speech therapist, over two mornings. The manual I received states the following:

- The criteria in developing Makaton as a communication 'language' was that it should be as pictographic as possible, to convey the meaning of the concept it represents
- It needed to be uncomplicated, so that the symbols could be drawn by hand if needed
- It needed to attempt to reflect language themes and structure
- The signs and symbols should reflect the multi-cultural society that we live in. [20]

There are Makaton tutors that put on courses that you can pay for privately,
if you do find for whatever reason that there is a shortage of classes in your area, or a long waiting list on the NHS.

Keys points:

1) It is important to speak the words whilst using the signs as the signs are there to support the spoken language, rather than replace it. Speak slowly and use facial expression to convey meaning, as it is a visual communication method which, whilst aiding memory, also focuses the child's 'looking and listening' skills. The signs are generally easy to copy, which only helps to reduce any frustration on the part of the child using it.

---

[20] The Makaton Charity, *Beginners Workshop Manual 1*, 2011, p.83

2) It is different to BSL as the word is also spoken.

3) Makaton doesn't have to follow the English 'spoken word' format e.g. you can say 'work I go' rather than 'I am going to work'.

4) Makaton is adaptable - depending on the child's ability to understand complex sentences, you can choose to only sign key words within a sentence, for example whilst saying 'Go upstairs and get your book and sit down on the sofa'. If the child is able to follow two signs and remember them in chronological order, they might sign 'book' and then 'sit down' whilst saying the full sentence. This also meant that Monty could learn to say his name by using the sign for 'M', rather than spelling out 'M-O-N-T-Y'.

5) On the written page, Makaton reads left to right on the page orientation. The symbols are often representative of the objects they represent.

It is important, if a child is learning to use Makaton, that the child's main care-givers also learn it (or the basics at least). We found when Monty started school that he was trying to use his signs to the teacher, who had no recent experience of Makaton, and she and I were worried that it might frustrate him that he was trying to communicate in this new way, and yet again, such as with his speech, he was not able to make himself understood. It was therefore seen as very important that the class teachers, teaching assistants and other support staff went on the basic Makaton course, and then they could also then teach the most relevant signs to the children within Monty's class. I felt it was important that not just one or two members of staff went on the training, as when Monty moved up a year we might have to start the process all over again. And, of course, having as many staff as possible in the school trained in Makaton would also benefit other children with any speech or communication difficulties, now and in the future.

I have also found Makaton useful when trying to get a message to my husband standing on the other side of a busy room - *What time are we going home? Can we leave now- I'm tired!* Very useful. A word of caution with siblings, however - I have often found Monty's older brother teaching Monty made-up signs, just to get in on the act! Do make sure you teach siblings and friends the correct signs from the beginning, too!

In case you were wondering, Makaton was developed in the 1970s, initially for the purpose of enabling deaf and cognitively impaired adults to be able to communicate using manual signs, by three people called **Ma**rgaret, **Ka**tharine and **Ton**y, hence the name. It has been adapted all over the world, for use in many countries.

British Sign Language (BSL)

British Sign Language is used as a fluent language by deaf people. The language has a non-spoken word order, with a unique use of grammar, and the use of some finger spelling for certain words or names. There are variations, like in spoken dialect and accent, depending on what part of the country the user is in. Facial expressions can also be used to convey emotion. As with the spoken language, different parts of the country have different dialects.

Signed Systems

In the UK, this represents 'Signed English'. The syntax and grammar used come from spoken language, and speech is used at the same time as signing.

This chapter at a glance

In this chapter we have covered some of the emotions that you are likely to experience after a diagnosis of verbal dyspraxia in your child, some of the healthcare professionals that you might come across now or in the future, research to keep abreast of when it comes to finding out what is happening in the medical world and alternative medicine, some alternative methods of communicating that involve signing to take the pressure off the child if they are becoming frustrated, and finally some of the speech therapy programmes available and the methodology behind them.

In the next chapter we will look at speech therapy in greater detail, including what to look for to ensure that you and your child have a great relationship with the speech and language therapist you are given (or choose), and some tips and guidance for things to work on at home, especially if you find yourself on a long waiting list for speech therapy.

****

Chapter 3

What to Expect in Speech Therapy

In this chapter we will look at what may be covered from the very beginning in speech therapy sessions; what to look for in a speech therapist to get the best for your child; the differences between choosing private speech therapy or NHS speech therapy, and the things that you can do at home to get the ball rolling in terms of preparing your child to learn the necessary techniques. We'll also touch on some of the frustrations that you may experience as a parent, in terms of waiting lists, the feeling that things are not going to plan, and the issues that may present in therapy from your child's perspective.

> ➤ **A parent's perspective**

Speech therapy can be an interesting subject. In some ways I think that whether or not your child will progress with their therapy and whether they will engage with the therapist doing it, is to a certain degree dependant on the personality of the therapist as well as that of the child. I have seen six speech and language therapists (SaLTs) work with Monty, and every one of them appeared to approach the therapy sessions differently. Some therapists seem to want to sit opposite your child, to enable eye contact, which also gives the impression of 'teacher and pupil' with a desk between them. Some sit by the side of the child, perhaps to avoid direct eye contact in the early days, and to encourage the child to feel at ease. Some have gone straight in to working on the Nuffield Centre NDP3 worksheets, asking for immediate copying and replication attempts of the sounds. Some have played with toys with Monty, almost in an attempt to convince him that he was not in a speech therapy environment, whilst still trying to elicit sounds such as animal noises. It really has been a mixed bag, and when the time has come for us to change therapists I have never really known what to expect each time we have walked into a new session.

I must admit, I did get bit worried in the early days in clinic, as we seemed to be spending quite a lot of our time on the mat, playing with cars and dinosaurs, but I came to realise that a SaLT can't just jump straight into a treatment plan without observing your child, and seeing what aspects of their personality they can pick up on; seeing what their coping strategy seems to be in the absence of clear speech, and also how they take to strangers. All of this is important in order to work out what the child needs, their strengths and weaknesses in speech and language, and how to take things forward in working out a strategy for speech therapy going forwards.

One of the things that worried me most in the early days was the thought that I was going to have to do much of the 'therapy' myself at home. It was clear that one half an hour session a week or fortnight was never going to enable Monty to get the practice and continuity that he needed to be able to learn and recall the speech sounds as the first step on the road to speech, so it would be down to me to help him - as his main caregiver, as I had given up my job to make sure that Monty got the help and time that he needed. Panic set in - I wasn't a qualified speech therapist! And yet I was supposed to go home and continue 'teaching' Monty myself, with a handful of worksheets full of pictures and symbols that were completely new to me.

Also, there seems to me to be a paradox in the way that learning within speech therapy is put forward to the parents. I remember being in clinic one day, where I mentioned that at home Monty and I had been working on a new sound - 'c' and 'ck' - as Monty had made some attempts to realise this sound accurately. Our speech and language therapist at the time said that I probably shouldn't be moving on to a new sound, as she herself hadn't heard Monty say it in clinic. At that point I felt quite frustrated when we got home, after thinking about it on the drive home. Monty only had speech therapy about every ten days at that point from the NHS therapist, and therefore the onus was on me, as his daily speech-work companion, to keep him going. If you weren't allowed to progress when you felt ready, and your child did not frequently have contact with the therapist helping you with the speech therapy programme, then were you supposed to halt progress until you next saw them? Not in our house, I have to say! I took the position that if I felt Monty was ready, and was periodically saying sounds that weren't in the folder, then I would add them to the folder at the back, and we would re-visit them at home when we had practiced all the other sounds at the front of the folder that the therapist had given us. In my opinion, just because Monty hadn't said something in the clinic setting, I wasn't going to let that hold him back, and our private speech therapist agreed.

So... what may be covered in the early sessions of speech therapy?

- Again, your child's history, from birth, including early speaking attempts and their feeding and drinking abilities as a baby up until now.
- The SaLT may look at your child's intention to speak – any sounds or words that they may make, any attempts at speech, and any mistakes included.

- They may observe your child's play, and social interaction.
- They may look to work out how many sounds (consonants, vowels and/or blends) that your child can do, as well as the length of any sentences, and whether the length and difficulty of the sentences affects the clarity and consistency of speech.
- They may try some of the sound cards of the NDP3 programme (if using) to see how your child responds to sound prompts, and whether they may respond to visual cues.
- They may keep a close eye on your child's understanding of words and language (receptive language). Can they follow simple instructions, such as 'Can you get the blue ball and put it in the red box?' or 'Which animal is the tallest? Can you sort these three animals in order, from big to small?'
- They may want to look in your child's mouth, to consider the muscle tone of the mouth, and internal movement –they may also check for tongue movement and possible tongue-tie (where there is a tight piece of skin between the underside of the tongue and the floor of the mouth that restricts the movement of the tongue.)
- They may touch your child's mouth and jaw in an attempt to model the correct position - this startled me at first for some reason, but it became really helpful to Monty to know what position his lips and tongue needed to be in to achieve the sound correctly.
- It is likely that the SaLT will take many notes for the writing of reports and therapy treatment plans for the next steps to be taken.

Points to consider when looking for a Speech and Language Therapist

Generally, I think there are the following points to consider, and in no particular order:

Membership of applicable bodies

Your speech and language therapist should be registered with The Royal College of Speech and Language Therapists (RCSLT). Private therapists may be registered with The Association of Speech and Language Therapists in Independent Practice (ASLTIP.) Practitioners must also be registered with the Health and Care Professions Council (HCPC.)

Qualifications

Speech and language therapists must be suitably qualified, which means that they must have been on a degree/post graduate speech and language programme, normally a three or four year course at a registered University.

Experience of verbal dyspraxia

Verbal dyspraxia is a specific speech disorder which requires a speech and language therapist with experience of it in order to effectively help your child. Not all speech disorders are the same, and they should not all be treated in the same way.

Experience with children with speech disorders

Some speech and language therapists have other specialisms, such as stuttering, or they may work with children with cleft palates or feeding difficulties. It is important that you have access to a therapist with experience and knowledge of speech and language disorders.

Cost - if looking for a private therapist

Speech therapy provided on the NHS will not need to be funded by you, however if you are looking for a private therapist, either in lieu of or as a top-up to NHS therapy, then make sure you establish the cost before embarking on a course of therapy. Depending on where you live, speech therapy costs are likely to be between £40-£70 per hour. If you have private healthcare, you may be able to reclaim some or all of the costs, so do check your policy.

Method of providing therapy

It is important to consider where therapy sessions will take place, the length of the sessions, and the intended frequency of the sessions. You need to know that you will be able to get there, or have the SaLT come to you, perhaps in your home. You will need to ensure that you know who will be attending, the parental involvement needed, what format the 'homework' will take, and what follow up the SaLT will undertake to assess progress and keep in touch with you, as the parent, and also with the other professionals involved in the care of your child.

I have to say, and this might be a personal preference, but I think one of the most important factors in looking at a speech and language therapist as an individual or as part of a general service, is to have a level of *consistency*, be that perhaps of the place in which the sessions take place, but most obviously in terms of the therapist that leads them. Some of the constant changes in Monty's provision have been unavoidable due to staff changes, and the lack of a constant therapist has seemed in the past to unsettle him quite a bit. I must say, though, that all of the therapists that I have met have obviously enjoyed their job, are very clearly set on helping each child that they work with as much as possible, and have been very keen to help Monty in the best way that they could.

> A Parent's Perspective

Monty has been assessed by two paediatricians, has seen five NHS therapists, and has one private speech and language therapist who has been helping us ever since we first knew that there was a problem with his speech. The reason for him seeing so many NHS therapists lies in the fact that there were staff shortages (resulting in a therapist being drafting in from another area), another left for a new job, and another moved cases. All were nice people, and obviously had Monty's best interests at heart, but the lack of consistency in the type and level of therapy, in addition to the constant change and time spent getting to know each new therapist, had a detrimental effect on Monty's confidence and progress in my opinion.

It took a little bit of time, but after talking to the head of the speech and language unit we were able to get our point across about the fact that we need regular therapy on *at least a* weekly basis, and from a consistent therapist. The manager of the area speech and language therapists (the same lady that had first diagnosed him, actually!) sat in on one of Monty's sessions, and I think that she could see that, for whatever reason, Monty had not progressed as much as we all would have liked. It was useful to have another extremely experienced therapist have a look at what was going on, and from this point on it was agreed that weekly sessions were needed, and in the school environment where Monty felt most comfortable having his sessions. If this taught me anything, it was to not give up when you feel that things are not quite going to plan, and to have the conversation with the right person who you feel can make the necessary changes.

Now that Monty has a settled routine of seeing his NHS therapist once a week and his private therapist one a week, and both in the school setting, which he has done for the last four months. I am sure that these changes are not a co-incidental contribution to the current level of progress that has occurred, and we now seem to have a level of consistency and balance, along with the in-school help, that we so badly needed over the last year or more.

NHS Provision for SLT

Generally, if your child has been referred to a speech and language therapist or clinic for assessment, and meets the criteria for the provision of speech therapy, then you should be offered some. There is no choice, to my knowledge, of a preference in who will be your therapist, as usually cases are allocated on a 'caseload by caseload' basis and you will be offered a place where one exists. The SaLT who assesses and diagnoses your child may not be the SaLT that you then are allocated to provide the therapy needed. The amount of therapy provided is often a given, depending on the area in which you live – some local authorities/Trusts in the UK may provide twice a week sessions, some once a week, and some a lot less, depending on the severity of the case of verbal dyspraxia and the availability of a suitable therapist. Hopefully you will get lucky!

There should be some things that you can have a say in, though – you should be able to have a say in where it takes place and who will be present. Also, don't be afraid to question why some things are suggested, how the therapy will take place, and for how long each block of therapy will be allocated. As always, a written diagnosis is always helpful in determining the type and length of speech therapy that will be necessary.

Independent Speech and Language Therapists

Independent therapists will have been through the same training as NHS therapists, but may choose to work all or some of their time as an Independent, or specifically within schools or other organisations. They should be members of the Association of Speech and Language Therapists in Independent practice (ASLTIP). All ASLTIP members are certified members of The Royal College of Speech and Language Therapists and are registered with the Health and Care Professions Council. You can use the database search on the website (www.helpwithtalking.com) to find an independent, registered SaLT in your area. The website states that:

'Independent Speech and Language Therapists will offer an initial consultation which will usually include an assessment (formal or informal) and a report setting out the findings. The purpose of this consultation is to ascertain the need for speech therapy and to gather information which will form a base-line for therapy. If speech therapy is required, the therapist will offer a series of speech and language therapy sessions which are specifically designed to meet the needs of the individual.'[21]

An independent therapist may use the NDP3 programme and other therapy programmes to provide speech therapy. Our independent therapist has used a variety of techniques and programmes with Monty, as one of the benefits of individual practice seems to be the freedom to do so. The variety of the sessions have always been one of the great things, and often Monty has found himself talking to a speaking frog, playing basketball where he had to 'dunk' the speech sounds, sitting in a cardboard boat 'fishing' for words, and making a spell 'soup' of words at Halloween. The sessions are always fun and entertaining, and Monty has got so much out of them.

---

[21] www.helpwithtalking.com (Retrieved December 2014)

Independent Speech and Language Therapy - how much does it cost?

It seems that this can vary quite greatly, depending on the type of SLT that you need, the area in which you live (the higher costs may be seen in London and surrounding areas), the experience and knowledge of the speech and language therapist (SaLT) you have chosen, and where the therapy is to take place (perhaps at the your home, your child's school, or in a clinic setting.) Make sure you ask about any extras that may come on top, for example, are travel costs extra?

I would suggest that you do your research - have a look at the websites of any SaLTs that are local to you, chat to fellow parents of children with verbal dyspraxia for recommendations- and maybe meet with a couple of therapists to see if you 'click'. The most important factor for us, more than the cost, was that we had confidence in the individual's ability, that they had previous experience of providing SLT to children with verbal dyspraxia as opposed to being more of a generalist, and that they were nice to be with! We were very lucky in that we really liked our independent SaLT from the very beginning; she came highly recommended, and we did not feel the need to look around, and we found her to be excellent with Monty from the very start.

If you have private health insurance then some or all of the fees may be covered. Make sure before you commit to a plan of therapy that you know exactly what will be covered by your insurance (and if there is a cut off-point), and whether the SaLT that you have chosen is recognised by the insurance company as eligible to provide the therapy you require. You may need to pay the fees up front, and then be reimbursed at a later date.

Should there be a preference for either an NHS or independent SaLT?

I don't think so. The most important things are:

- That you, and your child, find them easy to get on with. You could be spending many months or years with this person and they will most likely come to feel like 'part of the family.'
- That the person (or organisation) are able to offer consistent, regular therapy at an acceptable level as designated by the applicable professional bodies
- Waiting times! If, like us, you find that there is a long NHS waiting list, then it might be an idea to consider private therapy sessions, at least in the interim period. This of course depends on the severity of the verbal dyspraxia, and the means of paying for it.
- That the therapy happens at a time that is conducive to your child benefiting from it. We found that morning sessions worked the best for us, either during the week or at weekends. In the afternoon Monty used to fall asleep in therapy, especially when he was only three! Remember that the brain is a 'muscle' which tires easily, and sessions late in the day might not be suitable.

An explanation of some of the key terms you might hear used in speech therapy

Articulation: The way in which speech is produced; the ability to make clear and correct speech.

Auditory bombardment: The constant use and repetition of targeted sounds. For example, if working on the sound 's', there might be a sentence such as 'Simon was singing a song in the shower,' or the repetition of several words over and over – 'sand, sea, sand, sea' etc.

Expressive language: a way of communicating with others, primarily with speech but also with gestures.

Fricative sounds: These are long sounds, requiring continuous airflow through narrow constriction of the vocal tract, and include 'f', 'v', 's', 'z', 'th' and 'sh'.[22] In Monty's learning of phonics at school, he knows these sounds as 'stretchy' sounds (cue hands making a stretchy movement, as if pulling on a rubber band) which is quite a useful way of looking at it as the movement mimics the long sound.

Intonation: The change in spoken pitch that gives emotion and attitude. An example would be 'lifting' the end of a sentence to a higher pitch to indicate a question being asked as opposed to a statement or fact being made.

Phonics: How the letters of the alphabet actually sound, either individually ('t') or joined ('ck'.) Learning phonics is also one of the building blocks of teaching children to read and write, which involves the blending of sounds to achieve words.

Plosive sounds: Short sounds such as 'p', 't', 'k', 'b', 'd', 'g' , whereby the vocal tract is blocked and the airflow stops to create a quick, short sound. In Monty's learning of phonics at school, he knows these sounds as 'bouncy' sounds (cue miming bouncing a ball, in short sequence.)

Semantics: The meaning of language, and the relationship of words and sentences in the context of language.

Things to think about doing at Home
It may be that, like us, you have a bit of a wait between diagnosis and actually starting speech and language therapy, so in this section there are some ideas of things to try at home.

─────────────────

[22] www.speechandlanguagekids.com (Retrieved December 2014)

Organisations that can help

You might like to consider looking at the following organisations for information, guidance and help:

- Add-vanc
- Afasic
- I Can
- CASANA (Apraxia-Kids)
- Local SEN groups

Courses for Parents

There are various organisations and courses that are available for parents to go on to help you understand how to help your child learn to talk, and to get a better understanding of the building blocks of learning to speak. Elklan (www.elklan.co.uk) run a whole host of courses for parents, speech and language therapists and teachers to enable them to support the speech of the children in their care. One of the courses is called 'Let's Talk Under 5s' and I have found some of their worksheets very useful. Some of the downloads are available for free on the website, if you register your details.

The Elklan website lists the following outcomes as benefits of attending a course[23]:

- Understanding why children have difficulty learning to talk
- Know how to help a child understand what you are saying to him or her.
- Interact at an appropriate level with the child.

---

[23] www.elklan.co.uk/information/parents-and-carers/benefits-of-elklan-training (Retrieved December 2014)

- Know how to help a child develop his or her talking.
- Adapt the way you speak to the child so that they understand more of what is said.
- Supports a speech therapy programme that the child has been given to follow.

Financial help that may be available

Disability Living Allowance (known also as DLA) - is a social security benefit designed to help pay for the extra costs that having a disability entails. It is not means-tested and can be claimed on behalf of children. It can be useful for paying for different types of therapy, books, communication aids, day trips, and perhaps fun or educational activities to help your child. The Afasic organisation has produced a leaflet to help with applying for DLA called 'Claiming benefits for children with speech and language impairments' which is available on their website. You can apply for DLA via the government website (currently www.gov.uk), and there are various organisations that will help you fill in the forms, as well as the helpline.

Depending on your circumstances, you may also qualify for Carer's Allowance if you are the child's carer and meet the necessary criteria. The information on this is also found on the above government website.

Speech therapy aids to consider obtaining

- Things to aid blowing - straws (sucking and blowing through them) - drinking liquids, blowing feathers, blowing light footballs to play table football, even chocolate - Maltesers work well in our house!) Encourage blowing raspberries, even if it's in public places. Needs must! Blowing bubbles through a bubble wand, and blowing out candles (careful with the last one...)

- Things that make noises - duck whistles (very annoying after a while, but apparently very satisfying if you are the noise-maker!), harmonica, 'blow copter' (a mini helicopter blade that takes off into the air if you blow hard enough), party blowers, whistles, and slide whistles that change noise as you move the slider up and down.
- Things to aid licking movements – lollies, obviously, and ice cream. Try putting a small dollop of something sweet on the end of a lolly stick or teaspoon, and encouraging your child to lick upwards. There are also some tongue exercises called 'Mr Tongue' which you can search for on the internet – these revolve around a story of Mr Tongue who lives in your mouth and goes about his day (washing windows, for example) and each movement requires your child to copy it with their tongue.
- Monty's speech and language therapist sometimes uses a toy telephone that Monty speaks into and it carries his voice and plays it back to him in his ear which is great for auditory feedback.
- Some children may also benefit from some sort of movement whilst they are working on their speech, such as bouncing on a gym ball when doing therapy – it appears that the movement may stimulate some areas of the brain.
- Games - Flash cards used in phonics and early reading can be useful, and there are some sets that you can use to play snap or matching pairs. We also like to play bingo at home, as Monty has been able to say 'house' for some time, and could have a good stab at '(B)ingo' and 'line.' Counting games such as snakes and ladders are good, as well as games that require you to describe what you are seeing or drawing.
- Consider creating a 'talking book' which has pictures of all of the words that your child can say, including the names of family and friends. As you add more to the book, it can give confidence to both you and your child that new words are being conquered.

- There are many speech therapy apps that you can download, some of which are listed at the back of the book. You can search via Google or iTunes to find the latest apps. One thing I would mention is that a lot of the apps I have come across may have speech included with slightly different accents, and often the phonetic sounding of a letter or word can be different so watch out for that.

Getting organised
- Keep all of your therapy sheets in a folder, perhaps loaded from the back to the front so that the most recent sheets that you are working on are at the top. Put sounds or words that your child struggles with or has only just touched on in the folder, but in a separate section that can be brought out 'just for trying' as needed. Always good to be hopeful!
- Try working in short bursts, where you can just be with your child without any distractions. Get someone else to occupy any siblings, turn your mobile onto silent and turn the TV off. It can often help if your child actually initiates the activity - so be ready to drop everything on a whim! It might be that your child suggests a certain book or game, or speech therapy cards, or a certain sound to concentrate on. Make it something enjoyable, and remember to stop when they look like they've had enough.
- If you are reading with your child, remember to sit on their right-hand side so that if you are following the words with your finger at the same time, you are drawing their eyes across the page from left to right, and not covering up the words yet to come on the page.

Positive re-enforcement
- Through trial and error, I have come to find that there are different ways of saying the same thing, which are likely to give positive encouragement rather than sounding like a correction. Try to find a

different approach to saying 'No, that's not right - say it like this' if your child has made a mistake. I did a search on You Tube and came across many great clips of speech and language therapists in therapy sessions, and found that there were some great ways of correcting a wrongly-said sound or word. For example, if you say 'cat', and the child replies by saying 'nat', instead of telling them it is incorrect, you might try something like, 'I heard *nat*. Let's try *cat*. Can you say cat?' In this way, you are pointing out the word that you heard that was incorrect, and are modelling the correct sound again for the child to attempt to repeat.

- Congratulate the successes, and make a big thing of them, as long as this is what your child likes. I found that in the early days Monty was shy about his sound attempts, and if I made too big a deal of his great sound work then he was likely to hide behind his hands. Nowadays he is in to doing high fives all around the table when we get some good speech work!

- Also, it is important to try not to ask too many questions. Instead, it's good to concentrate on 'commentating' on what's happening. For example, instead of asking, 'What is that?' try saying, 'Oh look, it's a big orange giraffe.' This approach takes the pressure off the child who may be anxious about not being able to find the right words to answer you or make conversation; it eases into a conversation whilst potentially introducing some new words. By making an observation, and then hopefully eliciting a response, you are ideally avoiding getting a one word answer.

Take every opportunity...
- When you are out and about, or just going about your daily life, use everything you are doing as an opportunity to practice your sounds and words. Often the distraction of 'action' makes a child (and perhaps the adult, too!) forget that there is an alternative

purpose. Farms and zoos are great (try animal's names and their noises, sizes, colours)
- Supermarket shopping (great for counting, reading the shopping list, food identification)
- Sorting out cupboards (counting plates, sizes and colours, identifying things to go in piles that are the same or different, stacking)
- Walking in the park (count the trees and dogs, jump on the spot or do star jumps as you repeat sounds together)
- Driving in the car- (spot a particular colour car and shout the colour out, play 'I spy', play the A-Z game for all sorts of different subjects. For example, if it is about animals, the first person would say 'A for... anteater.' The next person would say 'B for... bat' and so on until you get to 'Z.' Watch out for 'Q' and 'X'!
- Concentrate on word patterns and rhymes, seeing if your child can add other words by recognising the parts of the word that cause the rhyme. An example would be cat, sat, mat, hat, rat and so on.

Learning through play, rather than just repeating sounds and words off cards seems to work best in our house. Anything including puzzles, playing snap, building with dominos, making dens, drawing pictures, or building with Lego is good with Monty.

Two steps forward, one step back...
Sometimes, for whatever reason, be it age, tiredness, choosing to take control, negative emotions towards therapy, despondence, or some other reason not listed, your child may decide they have had enough of speech therapy for a bit. Also, relapsing can happen. It happened to us after just a few months in to therapy, whereby we had a two week break and Monty lost all the words he had over Christmas period. In the wonderful book, 'Speaking of Apraxia – A

Parent's guide to Childhood Apraxia of Speech', the author Leslie A. Lindsay offers four suggestions[24] as to why this might happen:

- The motor planning and programming was not established correctly in the first place
- The 'linguistic complexity' of what the child is now saying (for example, longer and more complicated sentences) has increased above the child's current capability
- The child may not have fully understood the way a word is actually said, and therefore incorrectly thinks that an alternative word or pronunciation is the correct one,
- There may be actual underlying muscle weakness that might not have been detected before.

If you find that this happens to your child, try not to panic. Easier said than done, I know! I panicked a lot, and thought that I would never allow us to have a break from speech therapy again. However, slowly the words came back, and I think in hindsight that Monty was just deciding to have his own little break, in his own little way. For the record, we have had several little breaks from therapy since then, for example over the summer holidays, and it hasn't happened to us again. Talk to your speech and language therapist, and try to identify if there have been any triggers to the relapse, or if further investigation is needed into the underlying reasons.

---

[24] Speaking of Apraxia – A Parents' Guide to Childhood Apraxia of Speech (Leslie A. Lindsay, Woodbine House, 2012) pgs.355-356

Remember!

- Talk to your child as much as possible. You might think you sound a bit crazy by describing out loud what you are doing ('I'm washing up, and then I'm doing to sit down and drink a cup of tea. Cup of tea. See Mummy washing up the cup? That's for my cup of tea.' Don't be offended if everyone else in the house starts wearing earplugs.
- Learn how to imitate and exaggerate the mouth and tongue movements needed for the different speech sounds, as your child needs to be encouraged to look at you whilst you are talking and copy them accurately. It can often help to hold whatever you are talking about near to your mouth, so that the attention is fixed on your face (if the item is small, obviously!)
- Encourage eye contact, to ensure that social skills are included in a conversation. If a person isn't looking at us when they are talking, how do we know that they are talking to us? Also, I learnt in our speech therapy sessions that when Monty made eye contact with the person he was talking to, the louder his voice became. Often the absence of eye contact is linked to the child's low confidence in speaking, so any work in this area that you can do at home will be beneficial.
- Make a point of establishing what an outdoor voice and an indoor voice is, so that your child has an idea of what is an acceptable level of sound and noise. Some children with speech difficulties also have difficulty with knowing how to control their noise levels! Alternatively, if your child whispers, perhaps due to a lack of confidence, as with the above point ensure that they try to make eye contact to project their voice.
- Often it is deemed less imposing to sit next to your child, rather than opposite them when talking.
- All sounds made by your child are important, even if they don't make words or perfect sense. Practice makes perfect, and it is only

92

by constant attempts that your child will get there. There is some useful guidance produced by the Nuffield Centre entitled 'Advice sheets for Parents - Exercises to encourage your child to make sounds,' that your speech and language therapist should be able to provide you with if you are waiting to see a therapist.

And finally...

Speech therapy can be hard work. It can be boring, and repetitive, and annoying that other people around you are doing other things and don't have to go through it. Your child may not want to be there (there are parks to run in, and brothers to fight with!) so the more fun that you (and the SaLT) can make it, the better for all concerned. Make sure that your child is fed before you go, not hungry or thirsty, not too tired beforehand, and not distracted by various gadgets hanging out of your bag.

It can help if your child can realise that there is some reward for being there (I don't mean sweets, necessarily – but some kind of motivation that makes it worthwhile.) I have taken Monty out for lunch some days, or we've had a trip to the indoor play centre to let off some steam. Sometimes we've come home and cuddled up on the sofa to watch a favourite film. I think one of the main motivations can just be having some 'mummy' or 'daddy' time, and to just 'be'.

There are some things that you can do to make sessions a bit easier for everyone involved. Make sure that your SaLT knows your child's likes and dislikes. Our private therapist knows that Monty likes animals, and many of her activities include animals of some kind. Another therapist we once saw had a brilliant shark that randomly bit your hand when you counted its teeth– not to everyone's taste but Monty liked it! Let the SaLT know of any favourite pets and family members that your child is close to. Let them know if your child is feeling unwell, or is worried about anything. Perhaps you could let them take a favourite toy into the session with them. Monty used to take his bear in a suitcase, and bear would 'help' with the session by pointing to the Nuffield NDP3 cards. Whatever works, go with it!

****

Chapter 4

A Day in the Life...

In this chapter I shall be touching on some of the things in life that a child with verbal dyspraxia might experience at some point in time, both in terms of emotions, and also events and circumstances that may present themselves along the way. I hope that it both gives you comfort in the fact that your child may not be alone in some of their experiences, and also that there are some pre-used suggestions made that you might find useful in dealing with any situations that crop up. It certainly can be a rocky road at times, and there is no escaping from the fact that, for hopefully a short period in your child's life, they may have a slightly different experience in some elements of life than that of their peers. Try to remember that many of the issues touched upon will be transient, and often many of them can be apprehended with a good bit of pre-thought and pre-planning. Others may need a bit of humour thrown in for good measure, and the odd bit of 'biting your tongue' as a parent, especially to unhelpful comments and observations by others who have no idea what you and your child are going through!

> ➤ **A parent's perspective**

Although speech is a complex process when you break it down to its composite parts it is, generally, something that we all take for granted. We learned to talk when we were young, as a part of the automatic normal passage through toddler-dom, into childhood and then adulthood, and probably thought little of it at the time. For many, even learning to read, spell and write may have passed without little thought, as the necessary skills and techniques it required may have been easy to come by. Communicating with other people is one of the most basic and yet fundamentally important skills we need – it is how we make friends, how we get our needs met, how we tell others our emotions, even how we go about getting a job, a house, a partner. So when a child does not have that capacity, things can obviously get a bit worrying for all concerned, for now and for the future.

I found it useful to explain to Monty what his condition was from an early age, if only for the reason that I wanted him to know that *we knew*, as his parents, what his difficulties were in trying to speak, and that we knew how hard it was for him to cope sometimes. As a parent, I think it is quite easy to feel helpless when you can't immediately make things right for your child when something is wrong, and to feel that you are in some way letting them down. The problem can sometimes seem too big, especially when they seem to be struggling and aware of what is happening, and it can be hard to step back and take in the bigger picture.

Above all, it takes some time to realise that that your child is not defined by their condition – it is just something that currently sits with them, and they are moving towards the light at the end of the tunnel so to speak. Every speech therapy session at clinic is a step forwards. Every time you practice your sounds at home is another, as is the ten minutes you spend watching Mr Tumble, or singing the alphabet slowly on the way to school.

If only you knew...
I've often wondered what the world must feel like from the perspective of the child with verbal dyspraxia. There is a lovely document on the Apraxia Kids website (www.apraxia-kids.org)

entitled, *If I Could Only Tell You, I Would Say...,* which touches on some of the things a young child with verbal dyspraxia might say if they could, in relation to what might make them happy, scared or sad. There are also letters on the same site that parents can customise to give to new teachers, to explain your child's condition, and their likes, dislikes and needs, and how to get the best from them in the classroom.

Monty has, for obvious reasons, often found it hard to express his emotions verbally. This has in the past led to him compressing those emotions into pure frustration tantrums, where often nothing has been able to calm him down. It has also been difficult to determine how he feels about having verbal dyspraxia. A few things have come out over the past few months, little snippets of information, that have given us as parents an insight into his little, somewhat hidden, world. There was the one time when he told me, 'Mummy, me sad', after I asked him how he felt about trying to get his words out when he was struggling, that also made me feel so sad, and *cross. Why couldn't I fix this?* If I could feel this upset, I couldn't believe how Monty could cope with those types of feelings on a daily basis.

There was another time when we were travelling with another parent with a child of Monty's age, whereby the child leaned over and said to Monty, 'I don't like you.' Any other child might have retorted with a suitable insult, but Monty stared straight ahead, bolt upright, and from my position in the front of the car I could see the sadness in his eyes when I looked around, and my stomach twisted. It can be hard to know when to intervene, as kids will be kids and all manner of insults are thrown around with a carefree attitude in the playground, but it certainly brings out my more protective side when I know that it is hard for Monty to defend himself. I couldn't wait to get him out of the car and give him a hug. He seemed to be fine when we got to our destination, but I wondered later whether those moments stayed with him afterwards, and if they worried him.

Another time, when Monty was in nursery, we felt a little excluded from the rest of Monty's class. Everyone was friendly enough, except there was just one problem. We weren't invited to any of the other children's birthday parties. At first I thought it was just a co-incidence, and a case of different groups of friends within a wider group, until I saw invites being given out openly to the whole class, in plain view of us, but yet not to us. I think, thankfully, Monty was still too young to realise what was going on, but it hurt me to think about it too much, and I started to feel a little paranoid that we were being excluded. Of course, there may well have been other reasons for us not being included, but I think when your child is excluded you do start to think the worst. Throughout that year I came to find some lovely fellow mums that would go on to invite us on playdates, but that time was always a little difficult (for me, I think, not Monty).

Most recently, we were practicing the alphabet and Monty was doing really well, saying the letter names as well as the phonetic sound. When we got down to the letter 'U', I pointed to the picture beneath it, which was an umbrella. Monty said the letter, and then attempted to say umbrella. I asked him to try it again, and he sighed. In a stilted, broken sentence, he told me, 'I can't do it... with my mouth,' and whilst it was lovely to hear a sentence put together, in context and in the right order, it also made me realise that Monty knew it was his mouth that wasn't playing ball, and that he knew it was somewhat out of his control.

If only other people knew just how hard it is for those living with verbal dyspraxia, in pretty much every area of life!

Frustration Station

We have had periods during Monty's life when I lived each day, each waking moment actually, by walking on egg shells. During the 'terrible-twos' he used to get as cross as any other two-year old might, keen to escape the clutches of protective parents and have his own say about what he did and didn't want to do. And then, the 'frightful threes' set in, and Monty took it to another level. He was cross, for most of the day, and for the most part, at me in particular.

It might start in the morning, when I had struggled to work out what he was telling me about the food he wanted, where I had mistaken a request for 'water' (*ah ah*) for 'cornflakes' (also *ah ah*.) He would continue to feel cross when I would sing the wrong song he had been attempting to sing; when I picked the wrong coloured cup at snack-time, and when I had handed him the wrong toy from the pile stacked on top of the shelving unit that he had been pointing at. One frustrated little boy, and one equally frustrated (and exhausted) mummy. During this tough period, Monty would also lash out a bit, and his older brother used to bear the brunt sometimes, especially if the frustration related to the toys they were both playing with. Not a happy time for all involved!

Active, effective communication requires a speaker and a listener to both play their parts. The speaker needs to convey messages in a way that the listener will understand, and the listener actually needs to listen to be able to take in the message. If either cannot perform their part in a way that the other understands, then frustration is bound to set in (on both sides.)

Of course, we also communicate in many other ways, such as facial expressions, gesturing, general body language, and you might see that your child with verbal dyspraxia exaggerates their other ways of communicating. (Before Monty could say 'sad', and before he had learned the Makaton sign for the word, he used to cross his arms, shake his head whilst frowning, and grunt 'rrrrr' to convey this emotion.) If he was really sad, he would also stamp his foot! Of course, in the beginning I interpreted this as 'cross' and so when I said 'Oh, I see you are cross, Monty' this would often escalate into actual crossness (proper foot stamping!) because I had mis-read the situation.)

Some coping strategies with frustration and tantrums that our lovely speech therapist, Sue, gave me include:

1) Giving the child a choice, limited to two preferably, and with the choices on show so that a point with a finger is possible. I would always ask Monty to attempt the word in addition to pointing to the object. The conversation would go something like this: 'Ok, you have a choice of cornflakes or toast. Great, you want toast. Can you say, 'toast'.' I would accept an answer if Monty tried, to give encouragement, but if it was incorrect I would say, 'Yes, that's right, *toast*. Mummy will make you some *toast*.' Repetition is key!

2) Asking Monty to take me to show me what he wanted (for example from the playroom), if I couldn't work out what he'd said. If he pointed, again I would ask him to attempt the word, as I didn't want him to just rely on pointing and grunting to get what he wanted.

3) If the previous point hadn't worked, or if it wasn't possible to show me what he wanted, asking Monty if he could attempt the word again, or find another way to describe it to me. This could be where the Makaton sign for the object would come in handy.

4) Explaining to Monty that I understood that he was trying to tell me something, and that although I was working hard to understand, I couldn't work it out and that, could we try again in a bit? Sometimes this would work. I remember one time sitting on the stairs, cuddling Monty, with both of us in floods of tears. I said to

Monty, 'I'm so sorry. Mummy is trying hard to understand, and you are trying so hard to tell me what you want. Does this make you feel sad too?' He nodded, and it did help to calm things down a bit. I realised at that point in time, that by helping Monty to **identify** his own feelings, letting him know that I **understood** them, and in doing so saying that I **empathised** with him, often made him feel a bit better. I also pointed out the things that he was really good at, such as dinosaur noises, jumping, or riding his scooter.

5) Distraction. If the situation was really escalating, it was important to try to distract Monty from the thing that was causing the issue, and to try to quickly replace it with something else of interest. (On a tongue-in-cheek note - there is always chocolate if it's getting really bad...)

Disability and other labels

Verbal dyspraxia comes under the bracket of a special educational need (SEN), and is classed as a disability. As a family, my husband and I were unsure of this label at the start- it almost felt a step too far into a scary, unknown territory for us. I think that partly stemmed from the fact that to look at our son, he looks just like any other child running around the park, or playing with his toys. He has no physical problems; nothing that would make you feel that there were any difficulties when you look at Monty, until of course you heard him trying to speak. I also worried about the impact that such a label would have on Monty in other people's eyes. I remember several people asking me how Monty could technically be classed as disabled, when there was nothing wrong with him in physical terms.

However, I now feel that having a name for a condition can have its advantages. Firstly, you know what you're dealing with, and therefore that gives you some control over it by way of being able to research it, find out everything you can, and make informed decisions along the way. Secondly, it's not a fixed, unchangeable term, as hopefully in the future we may no longer need it as Monty will have overcome his verbal dyspraxia. Thirdly, having a correct diagnosis helps you to access the necessary care to successfully overcome the condition. And fourthly, it doesn't change the little person who has the label, nor does it 'become' them.

New people, and people-pleasing
Quite understandably, meeting and speaking in front of strangers, and even known family, can be a difficult experience. We have spent much of the last two years either avoiding certain situations (such as big birthday parties where Monty would be the centre of attention), or pre-empting how we would approach them (by avoiding busy times or busy places.) I have noticed over time that Monty has moved from flat-out defiance (*I will not talk to nor look at that man, no matter how much you coerce me!*) to being more of a pleaser, whereby he will say something, literally anything he can, in order to provide an answer.

Recently, we went to see Santa at a local farm during the run-up to the festive season. Last year Monty refused to talk to the red-suited, rounded and padded man in the corner, and instead hung back shyly. This year, when Santa asked Monty what he wanted for Christmas, Monty said 'iPad, please.' The jolly man laughed and raised an eyebrow at me, and we all giggled at the sight of a four-year old asking Santa for such an elaborate present. However, what Santa didn't know was that 'iPad' was one of Monty's newly-found words that he could say, regardless of what else he had written on his Christmas list. I knew that Monty wanted to provide an answer, and he used the words that he could in order to do so. In the short-term, that was great to hear, but in the long-term, I know I will need to be on the lookout to ensure that Monty doesn't just say what he thinks other people want to hear, or that he feels he has to answer with something, just for the sake of answering.

That's my friend... he doesn't talk

As a child with a speech and language disorder, I think there are some elements of making friends that will be difficult. I used to worry about the periods of isolation Monty experienced at nursery, when his teacher told me that he would take himself off to be alone, usually in the sand pit. Looking back, I think he probably found it exhausting to be trying to communicate at the pace required, and I'm not surprised that he needed some alone time to just be himself. At the time, though, as a parent, you don't want to hear that your child is by themselves, as you immediately tend to attribute that to them being 'lonely', even if that is not the case at all. I also used to worry about Monty's perceived lack of social skills, as he rarely made eye contact with his nursery friends and would talk over them with his babbles and grunts in the very beginning. I soon realised that children are very accepting, and his teacher explained that they took Monty and his attempts at communication as the 'norm'. One little girl used to tell him off for interrupting her, and used to say 'Wait until I've finished, Monty', which I actually found really sweet!

Over the last two years, Monty has managed to make quite a few friends who accept his speech difficulties, and now they don't really seem to notice it, which is lovely. If any new children comment on it, the questions rarely seem to last and are soon forgotten, especially if there is something far more exciting for them to be doing. I find that he often gravitates to the girls rather than the boys. Boys can be a bit more boisterous and loud, whereas the girls want to look after him.

I think it is really important to make a real effort to get to know your child's friends, and to organise plenty of playdates/social outings. If you are worried about going to another parent's house in the first instance, for example if you have concerns over whether the other child might be territorial over their own toys, then it might be better to do it on neutral territory.

We have always tried to give Monty an 'edge' that makes it easy for other kids to relate to, or to get a conversation going, so to speak. Monty's tree house that my husband built makes him the 'cool' kid in some children's eyes! Try to initiate interests for your child, such as swimming, child yoga, karate or musical instrument playing (anything that works on co-ordination or taxes the brain a bit is even better.)

Two final things. I had spent so much time thinking about how Monty would be perceived by the other children in his new class that it hadn't crossed my mind that the other children might feel worried by Monty's speech. One mum came up to me in the playground and told me that her child thought Monty was making fun of *her*, by making up a new language that she couldn't understand and be part of, as she couldn't work out why he would be talking differently than the other children. I was really pleased that this Mum had approached me, as I had no idea that other people's children might be feeling upset! I was then able to give this mum some information to help her explain to her child about why Monty spoke in this way, and then to give Monty's teacher the heads up that the other children in Monty's class might need some guidance to enable them to understand why Monty talks in the way in which he does.

Also, it has frequently concerned me that Monty couldn't necessarily tell me if he had been hurt or upset at something done to him at school. I had a word with his teacher to ask her to let me know if there were any issues in the day that I should be aware of, and we now have a home-school book kept in Monty's book bag that either we or school can write in if we have any concerns. It is always on my mind that I need to give Monty constant support in this area so that he continues to develop good self-esteem and self-worth. On the advice of a friend, I like to whisper little phrases or affirmations in Monty's ear before he goes into school to think about throughout the day – try something like 'You are Super Star Susie Smith and there is no-one else like you!' or even 'You were amazing at riding your scooter to school today – good job!'

Safety

Just think - what if a child with speech difficulties were to get lost? It doesn't bear thinking about really. I have always worried about Monty wondering off, and then not being able to tell an adult his name or who his parents are. To a certain extent, I would say that this has had an impact on where we have let him go without one of us as parents going with him, including parties, trips out, and even staying over at grandparent's houses.

As a basic precaution, I have liked to ensure that Monty had some form of identification on him if we have been going somewhere crowded or a to large place. I had a good look round for some ID bracelets on the internet that would be suitable for young children, and found a great selection of Velcro fabric ones on Amazon that are brightly-coloured and pleasing to kids. You can write the child's name and contact phone number in the inside and then wrap it around their wrist. There is also a spot for medical information and allergies if needed. I know some parents write on their child's arm in biro to do the same thing, but I always thought it better to put the information on a wristband.

I also bought a child's size high-vis jacket for Monty, which he wears if we are out at night or in winter, and try to ensure that we always have more than one adult keeping an eye out for him. It is hard, but it's natural to need to loosen the ties a little bit as children get older - play dates, trips to Grandad's house and 'no-parents-allowed' parties – but if you plan ahead and keep everyone in the know, and teach your child what to do in different situations, then things don't have to seem as scary.

We can't come, we've got speech therapy
Unfortunately, you can't be in two places at once. I always think it would be great to have one of those time-turners from *Harry Potter*, where you had the ability to go backwards and forwards in time, and like Hermione Granger catch up on all the things you missed by popping back into the past. However, in the absence of one of those, it is important to be super organised in planning where you need to be and when, and being realistic about what you can't fit in.

Therapy comes first in our house, even if it means that a speech therapy appointment means that we need to miss a scheduled football match on a Saturday morning (and football is important to the boys in this house!) Sometimes we have missed out on the things that other children have been doing. Sometimes we've come home from nursery or school and we've chosen to sit and work on our sounds, rather than go to the park or take up an offer of tea at a friend's house. It's hard, and sometimes you can feel a bit isolated and a bit of a bore – but you know deep down that you've done it for a reason and that the short term strain leads to long term gain. Putting in the time, even when it feels a bit inconvenient, is what it's all about.

Eating and drinking

Eating and drinking has never been a problem for Monty, but I know it can be for some children with certain speech disorders. There are mouth, jaw and tongue strengthening exercises that can be learnt to help with control when eating, which you should ask your speech and language therapist for help with if you find that this is a problem. If your child finds it distressing or embarrassing, try to limit eating in front of others where possible, or certain types or consistencies of food that exacerbate the problem.

Other people's perceptions

Ah, here's one of the tough ones. Other people's thoughts on your child's condition, their perception of their associated behaviour, and their ideas on how to relate to your child with verbal dyspraxia's speech can, in our experience, be one of the hardest aspects of the condition to deal with. It sounds silly, perhaps, as we can all develop a thick skin to what other people think about us, but when it is about your *child*, and about something that is totally out of their control, it is a hard pill to swallow. Below are a couple of examples of times when other people's actions or (re)actions, for want of a better word, have caused a variety of different emotions for us as parents, and the way in which we dealt with it. I'm not suggesting that these are the *right* ways to react, necessarily, just that this was the way we felt at the time. Sometimes a moment like those below can creep up out of nowhere, leaving you a little taken back – usually when things have been going well and you felt like normality had set in for the day!

> ❏ Not long ago, as a family the four of us went on a guided bush walk in a forest with lots of other families that we didn't know. The bush 'ranger' – a very nice man, and great with the kids that were

gathered around him (all eager to learn how to eat a mealworm and make nettle tea) — asked for help from some children near him to gather some wood. Monty was in his element, as kids usually are, being outdoors in the wild and having been asked to make a huge fire. He was chatting away, so caught up in the excitement that he didn't have any of his usual timid reservation in front of strangers. The ranger started to ask Monty a couple of questions about the wood, and Monty spoke back to him. The ranger then turned to us and said, quite innocently, and obviously thinking that Monty was a lot younger than he actually was, 'Sorry, didn't get that — I don't know baby talk.' Of course, our first thought as parents was that we hoped Monty hadn't heard him say that, and looking around the group of other parents it was clear to see that there was a level of embarrassment in the comment, as perhaps some of them had picked up on the fact that Monty had some problems with his speech. We didn't tell the ranger anything about Monty afterwards — he really was a nice man, and we didn't want to make an issue of it — but it was one of those times when something can cut through you like ice to the heart, and right when you least expect it.

❑ There was a time when we had a couple of people suggest to us that Monty was just being lazy, and that he would start to speak when he felt like it. Even though we had explained that that was not how a condition like verbal dyspraxia worked, the message just didn't seem to sink in. I didn't mind it if people didn't understand how the brain worked with the condition, or if they didn't understand what a diagnosis like that meant, but I couldn't bear it if they (so incorrectly) put it down to laziness. It seems in certain cases that if people can't understand an abstract idea or explanation, they tend to try to replace it with something more tangible that they can relate to.

❑ One another occasion, I took Monty out for lunch – just the two of us in a busy restaurant. Monty had just been at speech therapy, and his mouth was obviously nicely warmed up with all the exercises as he was chatting away to me ten to the dozen, about anything and everything, as he sat busily colouring in the kids menu. I suddenly felt eyes resting on me, and when I looked round to the table next to us where three women sat, mid-lunch, I saw they were all staring at us in silence. I ignored it to start with, but they kept doing it! Normally, at that point in time in Monty's development, you could see a look of confusion flash across people's faces, as you could see they were trying to work out if Monty was younger than he looked. It didn't help that he has always been quite tall for his age... After I felt they had been quite pointedly rude, even perhaps without meaning to, I decided to stare back, without saying anything. I wouldn't mind if they had asked what was going through their minds – just don't stare! And, I have to say, my actions did the trick as it obviously made them all check themselves, and they stopped staring...

There are many ways to explain to people what verbal dyspraxia is, and the problems that arise from it. I discussed some ideas for this in the **'What is Verbal Dyspraxia?'** chapter. However, it is also useful to have a few quick answers up your sleeve to the less helpful questions and comments, such as:

- 'apparently Einstein was also a late talker. Perhaps we have a genius on our hands!'
- 'He's just finding his feet in these new surroundings:'
- 'She's trying really hard, and making great progress.'

Short and sweet, and nipped in the bud early!

****

Chapter 5

Education

There have been a few changes recently in terms of the provision of additional help that either can or *should* be provided in the education setting, and also the way in which additional needs are perceived, planned for and integrated into mainstream schools, which can only be a good thing.

Children with additional educational needs in nursery, school and beyond are known as having SEN (special educational needs). The four key areas included are communication and interaction, cognition and learning, social, emotional and mental health, and sensory and/or physical needs.[25] Have a look at www.senmagazine.co.uk (a website and also a magazine) for updates on legislation and useful articles on coping with SEN, as well as detailed information on dyspraxia as an SEN. Also look at www.sendpathfinder.co.uk for legal documentation and updates. The key pieces of legislation include:

The Children and Families Act 2014

Part three of the above Act relates to children and young people in England with SEND.

---

[25] *Summary of the SEND Code of Practice: 0- 25 Years: October 2014,* NASEN, Chapter 6: Schools (retrieved November 2014 from www.nasen.org.uk)

There is a Special Educational Needs and Disability (SEND) Code of Practice which details how various organisations are to comply with the legislation. The definition within the Code of Practice as to what constitutes a SEND is as follows:

> '*A child or young person has SEN if they have a learning difficulty or disability which calls for special educational provision to be made for him or her. A child of compulsory school age or a young person has a learning difficulty or disability if he or she:*
> *- has a significantly greater difficulty in learning than the majority of others of the same age, or*
> *- has a disability which prevents or hinders him or her from making use of facilities of a kind generally provided for others of the same age in mainstream schools or mainstream post-16 institutions.*'[26]

The Code of Practice contains information on how early identification and assessment aims to provide children and young people (aged 16-25) with SEND with the help and assistance that they need, to assure them and their parents of what reasonable service they can expect to have provided. It sets out how parents and children can expect to be consulted and involved about decisions on the support they receive, and the outcomes in life that

---

[26] *Special Educational Needs and Disability Code of Practice: 0-25 years – Statutory guidance for organisations who work with and support children and young people with special educational needs and disabilities* (Department for Education, Department of Health, July 2014) p. 15/16

they wish to see, such as further education and employment. The Code of Practice is statutory guidance for organisations such as local authorities, schools and NHS Trusts, and means that these organisations must fulfil their statutory duties contained within the Code of Practice, and be able to demonstrate that they are doing so, and how.

The main points to know include the following, which are different to the previous legislation of the SEN Code of Practice 2001[27]:

- It covers the 0-25 age range, and also includes guidance relating to disabled children and young persons, as well as those with special educational needs (SEN)
- There is greater parent and child/ young person participation in making decisions at a personal level, and also at a strategic level in terms of planning
- There is a focus on improving outcomes, in particular in terms of success in education and confidence in adulthood to pursue career and fulfilling life ahead
- There must be close co-operation and joint planning between the education sector, local health services and social care provision
- Local authorities have to publish a 'Local Offer' which sets out the general provision for 0-25 year olds with SEN and disabilities

---

[27] *Special Educational Needs and Disability Code of Practice: 0-25 years – Statutory guidance for organisations who work with and support children and young people with special educational needs and disabilities* (Department for Education, Department of Health, July 2014) p. 14

- The lead-in period for eventual replacement of School Action and School Action Plus in terms of the necessary support for pupils in the educational setting
- A new EHC Plan (Education, Health and Care Plan) which replaces Statements of Special Educational Needs (usually known as a 'statement.') The EHC Plan is usually considered when the needs of the child or young person are more complicated or complex than that which the Local Offer would provide.

The Special Educational Needs and Disabilities Regulations 2014
These Regulations set out in greater detail the process of how an EHC Plan assessment should be undertaken, the responsibilities on the local authority to abide by the strict timescales for notifying those involved as to whether an assessment will or will not be undertaken, and their reasons for doing so. It also details the information, advice and recommendations that should be sought for the undertaking of the assessment, such as from the parents, speech and language therapists, the child's school, any medical intervention, social care, and the input of an educational psychologist as necessary. They include information on the review process, and timescales and deadlines for actions.

The Regulations set out the way in which the EHC Plan should be set out.[28] An EHC Plan includes the following sections which may or may not all be filled in, depending on the child and the circumstances:

---

[28] The Special Educational Needs and Disability Regulations 2014 (12.1)

Section A:	The views, interests and aspirations of the child and his parents or the young person
Section B:	The child or young person's special educational needs
Section C:	The child or young person's health care needs which relate to their special educational needs
Section D:	The child or young person's social care needs which relate to their special educational needs or to a disability
Section E:	The outcomes sought for him or her
Section F:	The special educational provision required by the child or young person
Section G:	Any health care provision reasonably required by the learning difficulties or disabilities which result in the child or young person having special educational needs
Section H1/H2:	Any social care provision which must be made for the child or young person as a result of any other social care provision reasonably required by the learning difficulties or disabilities which result in the child or young person having special educational needs
Section I:	The name of the education establishment that the child or young person, and/or parents have requested be named on the Plan.
Section J:	Personal budget statement for funding with specific outcomes
Section K:	Advice gathered to form the basis of the information in the plan.

It might look like all this makes for a large document, but in reality Monty's EHC Plan is only nineteen pages long, and the majority of pages within it contain the reports written by the professionals consulted such as the SaLT, Educational Psychologist and the Paediatrician.

The Special Educational Needs (Personal Budgets and Direct Payments) Regulations 2014

In some situations, you may be able to ask for a personal budget whilst the draft plan is being drawn up, or during a review after being awarded an EHC Plan, which helps with securing the provision of goods and services which are perhaps individual to the child, and not part of the general local provision. It does appear that the local authority in each area can set out the terms as to when a personal budget can be requested and for what reason – in our area it does not include educational provision and only looks to include provisions under health and social care, so do read up on your local offer (search the internet for your district/ local authority's pages on disabilities and local provision) to see what is intended to be included in your district.

I had hoped that the top-up speech and language therapy that we pay for privately could be covered by a personal budget, but that was not the case where we live.

Equality Act 2010

The Equality Act 2010, in relation to the topics covered here, looks at ensuring that no discrimination is given to children and young persons with SEND by schools in respect of their admissions policy, and that equal rights are established throughout all processes.

Note: All of the legislation discussed here can be found in full at www.legislation.gov.uk.

Statements and EHC Plans

As of September 2014, the old-style statements are being replaced by the new EHC Plans. If a child has a statement already, they will usually be converted to the new EHC Plan at their next review, and in any case, under the transitional arrangements all statements will need to be converted by April 2018.

Key information about EHC plans:

- AN EHC Plan is a legal document, which sets out what provision must be made for a child with SEN, and how those needs are to be met by the various services
- The plan goes through the process of the child's educational, health and social needs and what provisions need to be in place to meet those needs, consulting those who have an input into the care of the child.
- The Local Authority has to make a decision as to whether or not to issue a Plan (if they choose not to, you are entitled to appeal to the Special Educational Needs and Disability Tribunal for your area – this must be done within two months of receiving the decision- guidance can be found at www.gov.uk under the SEN pages, or via National Parent Partnership Network (nppn@ncb.org.uk))
- The process must take no more than 20 weeks from start to finish.
- If they agree, they will issue a draft plan which you get to comment on, and name the school of your choice if needed.

- You will then be issued with a final plan, of which the local authority has a legal duty to ensure that the educational provision is delivered.

➢ A Parents Perspective

It was while Monty was at nursery that the subject of getting a (then) statement of special educational needs was introduced. I wasn't sure whether we needed one, as I had great faith in the school that I knew Monty would be going to. However, it was his teacher who decided, on the basis of his IEP (see below in the section entitled IEP for more information on this) that it would be in Monty's best interests going forwards to apply for one. I think it was a lack of certainty at how he would cope at school, coupled with the severity of his condition and the slow progress that he had made within his nursery year, that really made the teaching staff suggest it. Also, we knew that if we wanted Monty to attend a specialist speech and language base, in our area he would not be able to do this unless he had a statement.

We found the process to be quite straightforward, even though it was new in our area and the council had not been through the process many times before us. We actually ended up becoming part of a group who trialed the process in our area! After all of the necessary reports had been collated from the professionals involved in Monty's care, and we had written our own supporting statement which included our concerns for Monty's future, his difficulties in communicating and how this affected his daily life, the application was sent off. Not long after (and the first application was actually lost in the process, causing us to re-send!) we heard that our request for an assessment had been upheld. After that, we had a meeting with members of the SEN staff from the council that were responsible for putting the plan together, along with the

118

professionals who had written the supporting reports. Everyone around the table had an input into what the plan should actually say, and how the outcomes should be achieved. I have to say that the paperwork seemed a little lengthy, but when the draft plan arrived it wasn't that long at all - in fact it was quite concise. Once we, as parents, were happy with the plan, the final plan was received by us and the school within about three weeks, and the school were then duty-bound to fulfil the information contained within it in relation to Monty's learning and access of the curriculum.

Monty's EHC plan currently includes four outcomes that we jointly agreed for Monty, involving his ability to communicate with his peers and adults in order to tell them his needs and wants, to enable him to have a wide group of friends to sustain good relationships, to enjoy and have confidence in his learning and to make progress in line with his age and ability, and to enjoy all aspects of his school and family life. The outcomes are quite general, but it is within the sections entitled *'What will the short term targets be?'* and *'What will help Monty achieve this outcome and who is responsible?'* and *'How will we know the outcome has been achieved, and what are the arrangements for monitoring this?'* that the detail is available to see how the plan fits together.

Common Assessment for Families (CAF)

Where there is a need for many different organisations, agencies and services to be involved with the care and planning for a child, sometimes a Common Assessment for Families (CAF) is a process that is used. It aims to provide a method for assessing the needs of children and young people to support earlier intervention and to improve joint working and communication between services. It uses a common language for assessment purposes thereby giving a more consistent view of what the child needs, and it improves the coordination and consistency between assessment, hopefully leading to fewer and shorter specialist assessments.

IEP (Individual Education Plan)

An IEP is an Individual Education Plan that is written for a child with SEN that details the extra things that a child may need in order to access the curriculum and make the progress that they need to. It details the plan for progression, aims to monitor the effectiveness of teaching, include the additional support needs that are to be provided from within the school, allows for the inclusion of the parent and involves the parents and the child in the child's learning and the identification of specific targets. Monty even had one from the age of 18 months, and it was a useful plan that listed where he was falling behind and the actions that needed to be taken by his nursery to support him.

If you have an IEP or several of them collected over time, make sure that you keep copies of them as they are useful to prove that the verbal dyspraxia has been an on-going condition that has required changes to be made for your child in relation to their education, which is useful if you later find that you need to apply for an EHC Plan assessment. Do bear in mind that all speech targets, in relation to an IEP and an EHC Plan, should be devised in line with SMART properties, i.e. they should be Specific, Measurable, Agreed and Achievable, Realistic and Time-based.

Exceptional Needs Funding (ENF)

You might find that your child's nursery or school apply for something called Exceptional Needs Funding, which can sometimes be granted by the local authority to help with additional costs of support and resources where it has been deemed by a panel of professionals that a particular child has complex, exceptional needs that are substantially over and above that of other children of the same age.

The role of the SENCO

A SENCO is a Specialist Educational Needs Co-ordinator that works in a school, and is the person responsible for the day-to-day operation of the school's SEN policy. All mainstream schools must appoint a teacher to be their SENCO. They will also co-ordinate any additional support needed for pupils with SEN and liaise with their parents, teachers and other professionals. The SENCO has responsibility for requesting the involvement of an Educational Psychologist if needed, and works primarily to ensure that there are no barriers to the learning and integration into the school for children with SEN. The SENCO may be the person who formally requests an ECH Plan assessment, in conjunction with the parents of the child, and will be present at the EHC Plan meeting.

Educational Psychologist

The Educational Psychologist looks at whether a child or young person needs any additional help if they are struggling in the educational environment or experiencing problems with their emotional and social well-being as a result of any problems they are facing. They will consult with other professionals involved to advise on the best approaches and provisions to support learning and development; they can help with behaviour management programmes; they can give advice on how to adapt classroom learning to help those with SEN, they can assist with developing and applying effective interventions to promote psychological wellbeing, and they look to raise educational standards for those with SEN.

Our Ed Psych, as they can be known, came into Monty's nursery and looked at how his communication difficulties presented issues for him in the class environment, and whether or not she thought he was coping ok. She introduced some strategies to get him further involved in the class as a group, and how to (at the time) manage any frustration issues that he had at home.

What a school might do in relation to needs of a child with verbal dyspraxia

- Introduce social skills training, such as 'taking turns' and making eye contact via games. Concentrate some learning into small groups, so that the environment does not seem so 'scary' for a child with a condition like verbal dyspraxia, whereby large classes can seem off-putting in terms of speaking out loud in front of others
- Ensure targeted speech practice throughout the day, often that the whole class can benefit from (think of phonics work, which all children in Reception and Year One would be doing anyway.)
- Enable the teacher or Learning Support Assistant (LSA) to undertake one-to-one help with a child, perhaps in reading, writing, maths or literacy
- Give all children the chance to talk in class in a situation in which they feel confident. For example, if a child with few words had most of their words that they were able to say in one given subject, to allow that child to do 'show and tell' on that subject. Monty has taken in some of his drawings from

home to show his class, and whilst I have told his teacher in advance what they contain in case it wasn't clear at the time, Monty has managed to get his point across because the subject matter was personal to him and something he knew well. This sort of practice can really help to build confidence in public speaking.

What you can do in preparation for starting school
Knowing full well that we were 'up against' it, the following is a list of things we aimed to do for Monty before he started in his reception year at school (age 4/5):

- We helped him to learn how to hold a pen - Monty often swapped hands with pencils and pens, and didn't seem to favour a dominant hand for some time. We really worked hard on his grip and control, mostly by doing colouring, and eventually he emerged as left-handed.
- Tracing letters, shapes and numbers
- Help with recognising the alphabet, letter names and phonic sounds
- Playing snap, and memory games such as matching pairs
- Labelling **all** of your child's things (I even labelled Monty's socks!) to avoid anything going missing that needs to be asked for.
- Take full advantage of all settling-in sessions to accustomise your child to their new environment, including the staff they will see, and show them where everything goes (such as name pegs, coats, water bottles, and wellies etc.).
- Taking advantage of playdates with new classmates in the summer holidays
- Unless your child will be eating a packed lunch, get hold of a

copy of the school dinner menu and show them how it works in terms of choices. We also got to have a school lunch on one of our settling-in days, which really helping in terms of showing Monty where he had to queue, where to sit, and where to clear his tray.

- Discuss with your child's new teacher how they intend to let your child answer in class. For example, when answering the register in the early days, Monty was allowed to say 'Yes' or 'Mmm' for his name, whilst doing the Makaton letter for his name. As long as he made a good attempt then that was acceptable, and his teacher would finish his name off for him by modelling the sound or word.

What type of school?
We faced a tough decision just before Monty started school. Should he attend a mainstream school, the one that his older brother attends and the place he has spent two years being told that he will one day attend, or could it in fact be in his best interests for the future to attend a special school that specialises in speech disorders?

I did some research, and found that there were a handful of 'speech and language bases' in our area, mostly attached to mainstream schools that had an allocated number of spaces for children coping with severe speech and language disorders. I made a few phone calls, and immediately some bases within travelling distance were out of the question as they only took children from Key Stage Two onwards (i.e. age seven and above.) I also knew that we didn't have an immediate choice about applying for a place, as we didn't have a Statement of Educational Needs or EHC Plan in place, but we wanted to have a look around one base that came highly recommended. We were advised by our speech and language therapist to go and see it, and I'm glad we did. I figured it was worth looking into, if only for the fact that you are really only able to make an informed decision when you are in possession of all the facts and choices available.

The base looked great – the teachers looked lovely, the school was friendly and welcoming, and when we arrived an assembly was taking place, with part speech, part Makaton, and as the children were singing (both from the main school and the speech and language base) they were also using Makaton signing. We found out that Monty would see a dedicated SaLT three times a week, and that children generally made good progress through Key Stage One. It all sounded good. However, there was one thing that stood out for us – that the base and the environment *didn't suit Monty's personality*. He is outgoing, sociable, and sometimes quite loud, and the classroom, with only a handful of children in it, was so quiet and still. I also noticed that not all children were following the same stages of the curriculum, as the base had children of reception age, plus also Year One and Year Two in it, so it didn't really have a classroom feel whereby everyone was involved with the same activities. We felt, on reflection, that we wanted Monty to be part of a busy classroom, whereby his social needs would be met, and his brother was in the same playground at lunchtime. We also felt that Monty would benefit from being around his peers that were talking at age-appropriate levels, which might somehow spur him on to work on his own speech in order to communicate with his new friends. Even though the condition of verbal dyspraxia doesn't work like that (if only!) we still felt that that was an important factor in his daily life at school.

On a small aside, the fact that the base was not in our town and was a thirty minute drive away also made me worry. School would be a taxi ride away, and if Monty was given a place it was likely that a chaperoned taxi service would be included. At the time he was three, and I have to admit that the idea of putting my little boy in a taxi with people I didn't necessarily know, sending him off on the motorway filled me with dread. I have friends who do it for their children, and they assured me that I would get used to it, but it just didn't feel right for us, especially with Monty (at that time) unable to speak, and not yet even four.

Hindsight is a great thing, and sometimes it shows that it is worth it to give things a go, whatever the choice may be that you have to make. What was right for us won't be right for every family, or for every child, and thank goodness that we have these amazing bases and special schools that do such fantastic speech and language teaching for our children. We chose to give mainstream schooling a chance, as it felt right for Monty – although with a caveat that we could change our mind if needed- and so far I know that we have made the right decision at this point in time. If you find yourself in this tough position, remember that only **you** as parents can make that decision – no one can tell you which type of school you should send your child to - so make sure that you give yourself the time and space to consider all of the options, to work out what is best for your child.

****

Chapter 6

A Difference in Opinion?

For many months now, it has struck me as strange that there appear to be so many differences in the approach to overcoming verbal dyspraxia in the USA and the UK, yet the disorder is no different in terms of diagnosis and the necessary treatment. Why is this, I wonder?

One of the main areas of apparent difference lies in the definition of 'intensive therapy.' In Leslie A. Lindsay's book, *Speaking of Apraxia – A Parent's Guide to Childhood Apraxia of Speech,* the author writes that children with CAS (Childhood Apraxia of Speech, as it is known in the USA) 'need frequent, intense 1:1 therapy – at least in the beginning.'[29] She goes on to say that some speech and language therapists recommend at least two sessions a week, depending on the age of the child, the severity of the speech disorder and the ability of the child to concentrate, along with the time and money available on the part of the parent/carer. So that's a suggestion of two sessions a week – and don't forget that here we are talking about speech and language therapist-led sessions – not including the additional practice required at home.

It is very difficult to find a definition of 'intensive' speech therapy and what that actually means here in the UK. If you do an internet search on the topic, very little information is available.

---

[29] Speaking of Apraxia – A Parents' Guide to Childhood Apraxia of Speech (Leslie A. Lindsay, Woodbine House, 2012) p.121

One paper of interest that I have come across, however, is below:

RCSLT POLICY STATEMENT: DEVELOPMENTAL VERBAL DYSPRAXIA
(The Royal College of Speech and Language Therapists, 2011,
Retrieved on 14.12.14 from
www.ndp3.org/documents/rcslt2011dvdPolicyStatement.pdf)
This policy statement document from the Royal College of Speech
and Language Therapists states that
*One in six children is referred to local Speech and Language Therapy
Service and almost 40% of these have a primary speech difficulty,
also classed as Speech Impairment.'* It goes on to say that *'very few
presentations resolve without Speech and Language Therapy
interventions.'* The document says that *'specific evidence based
guidelines cannot be produced until more research is conducted'* and
*'DVD features can be present to any degree from mild to severe, and
have increasing impact on individuals as the demands of
communication increase. As its presentation may change over time,
additional challenges may arise. It may be that those progressing
from a severe to a mild difficulty are those who have responded to
therapy input; unfortunately there is insufficient data to determine
this at the current time.'* The report also states that the primary
objective of speech and language therapy in the UK lies in the
*'provision of the relevant amount and duration of direct SLT
intervention, planned, at times undertaken by, and at all times
coordinated by a specialist SLT. This need will vary over time and
between individual children, and the nature and intensity of
provision should be adapted to meet these varying needs and the
growing evidence base.'*

One of the most interesting points the report makes is that
*'there is currently variation of access to specialist SLTs across the
UK'*, with some areas identified as having no specialist speech and

128

language therapists with significant knowledge and experience of speech disorders such as verbal dyspraxia, as well as the fact that the report mentions the ASHA Research paper of 2007 (ASHA Technical Report on Childhood Apraxia of Speech (2007, www.asha.org)) highlighting the point that *'since children with DVD need repetitive planning, programming and production practice, they suggested that children need:*

- *Individual (rather than group treatment, delivered intensively (i.e. 3-5 treatment sessions per week with SLT)*
- *More frequent short sessions are preferred to less frequent longer sessions.'*

In relation to the above point, the report also quotes clinical experts in the UK that have suggested that *'some UK SLT services favour 'blocks and breaks' of therapy, e.g. 6 weeks therapy followed by 6 weeks consolidation period; others favour a consultative or advisory provision – this is contrary to the recommendations listed above* [of the ASHA report] *which are upheld by RCSLT as there is no robust evidence for these models of delivery at the time of going to press.'*

It would appear, therefore, that experts in this country uphold the suggestion that frequent therapy of several sessions a week is key to improving the condition, yet it seems anecdotally that this falls down when it comes to the actual provision of the therapy in some local areas.

If you can, have a look at the journal section entitled *Speech Therapy for Apraxia: Frequency, Intensity, 1:1* on www.apraxia-kids.org (Childhood Apraxia of Speech Association, 2003 – retrieved December 2014.) There are some interesting articles listed, mostly from the USA - some of the key points of which are listed below:

'Regardless of the primary deficit, children with severe speech impairment need intensive speech therapy early on. Young children benefit from frequent shorter sessions (e.g., up to four times/week for 30 minutes each session). These are preferable over longer, less frequent sessions.'[30]

'Although there are differences in definitions of intensive remediation for children with CAS, there appears to be emerging consensus within the literature that therapy should be conducted at least three to five times weekly, in sessions lasting between 30 and 60 minutes each, and that the intervention should be conducted on an individual basis.'[31]

'We recommend **therapy as intensively and as often as possible**. *Five short sessions (e.g., 30 minutes) a week is better than two 90-minute sessions. Regression will occur if therapy is discontinued for a long time (e.g. over the summer).'*[32]

---

[30] Skinder-Meredith, A. *Differential Diagnosis: Developmental apraxia of speech and phonologic delay.* Augmentative Communication News; 14 (2 & 3), December 2001 (retrieved from www.apraxia-kids.org/library/speech-therapy-for-apraxia-frequency-intensity-11, in December 2014)

[31] Penelope K. Hall, Linda S. Jordan, Donald A. Robin, *Developmental Apraxia of Speech: Theory and Clinical Practice*, 2nd Edition, page 200, Pro-ed Publishers, Texas, 2007. (retrieved from www.apraxia-kids.org/library/speech-therapy-for-apraxia-frequency-intensity-11 in Dec 2014)

[32] Shelley L. Velleman, Ph.D., CCC-SLP, Developmental Verbal Dyspraxia, Apraxia-Kids Website (retrieved from www.apraxia-kids.org/library/speech-therapy-for-apraxia-frequency-intensity-11 in Dec 2014)

The message pretty much across the board in the USA is that the more frequent the therapy, the better the prognosis – and this frequent therapy should be **at least** one or two sessions a week, with no long breaks between sessions. It also seems that speech and language therapist involvement is key – they need to establish the plan, provide the resources, keep things on track, pick up on any issues (for example with pitch, and breath control) and where things might need more input. For example, I didn't realise that Monty was 'sucking in' his 'f' sounds, rather than forcing the air out. It was a subtle difference, but one that was noticed and picked up quickly by his SaLT and which needed practice to rectify to establish the correct motor plan, which is something I think I might not have noticed for some time if his speech therapy was centred around us just doing our bit at home. Not only are qualified SaLTs looking at all of the above in relation to production of speech, but they are also interested in ensuring that this develops into clear, spontaneous communication which takes extra work to take things to the next level. Verbal dyspraxia is a complex condition, where not all features present at the same time, and it takes a knowledgeable, suitably experienced SaLT to keep an eye on where things are heading.

Another important factor that certain information originating from the USA suggests is important is that it is **imperative** to get help as soon as possible, if you have any concerns about your child's speech. Personally, in the UK I have experienced quite a bit of a 'wait and see' attitude in relation to some of the professionals involved, but as the Apraxia Kids website points out, waiting until school age to seek help might leave the child at a disadvantage, being that they have enough to be getting on with in terms of writing, reading, maths and social relationships. Also be aware that in the UK it appears that often parents are told, from information given to me from other parents I have spoken to, that they would be given 'blocks' of speech therapy, followed by breaks where they were signed off from therapy to allow for the family to work on speech work at home and to let it 'sink in'. This obviously depends on the individual child, their diagnosis and severity, but I know that in our case this would have worried me as any breaks in Monty's provision seemed to have a detrimental effect on his speech in the early days of therapy.

Anecdotal evidence, and personal experience on our part and that of many others I have talked to in the same boat, would suggest that in many parts of the UK, you would be unlikely to get more than one session a week provided by the NHS. This means that, if like us, you are offered one session on a weekly basis, you would likely be offered a 30 minute time-slot, with perhaps roughly 20 minutes of actual speech work allowing for note writing, general questions from the parents, and any reluctance or slow start from the child. It would suggest therefore, that home practice and that which takes place within the education environment (often by persons with no speech therapy prior knowledge or qualifications) is seen as the main way of upping the frequency of practice.

We asked over many months for more help, with a view to obtaining two sessions a week, but to no avail – the reason given that it was not policy to offer more than one therapist-led session per child per week, across the board. We felt, however, that staff shortages and cutbacks might have been a contributing cause to our requests being denied. I also knew that in other parts of the country, including several boroughs in London, it was common to see a child with severe verbal dyspraxia being offered twice a week sessions. We began to feel that our best hope was to aim for a guaranteed weekly session with a consistent SaLT, to continue to pay for the private sessions we had come to rely on so greatly, and to know that when the EHC Plan came into play, that we would be given the help in school with daily concentrated practice.

The other main difference across the pond seems to be the amount of information available, the process of getting the message out there, and the known and publicised research into the causes, prognosis and treatment approaches relating to verbal dyspraxia. You only have to do a quick search on the internet about the research and information resources available to see that the vast majority are US-based. I am of the opinion that in the UK we need definitive studies on the outcomes for children with verbal dyspraxia, to ascertain the most efficient speech therapy programmes and interventions, and a clearer understanding on the potential benefits of a clearly defined position of what intensive speech and language therapy can, and *should*, mean. Let's get the message out there!

****

Chapter 7

The Family Unit

This section is about the impact that a diagnosis of verbal dyspraxia might have on the family of a child living with the condition. I think the natural instinct is for the attention to be centred on the child that has been diagnosed, but I have come to realise that siblings of that child may also feel that there is some impact on their own lives and emotions, as well as the parents and wider family unit.

As a parent, you might find yourselves as the main person responsible for helping your child to get through this. We've discussed some of the emotions you might be feeling in Chapter 2, however after you've worked through any of these that you might have been feeling, the verbal dyspraxia is still there to be dealt with, and that has an on-going impact on everyone close to the child.

As a family (in whatever format or set-up that means for you) I think it is important to communicate how you are feeling to each other, and also to share with the family what is happening at each stage of the condition. If siblings are mature enough to understand, maybe let them sit in on a therapy session to see how it is for their brother or sister. Have a meeting that everyone attends, maybe at the kitchen table or out at a restaurant, where everyone gets to have their say (verbally, or via the use of an alternative communication system as appropriate) on any problems that are being experienced at home, or at school. Try to establish a common feeling that 'we are all in this together.'

Not long ago, I had to make a decision about how I, and we, were going to get this nightmare of a situation resolved for Monty. I chose to take a career break – I knew there was something wrong with his speech, my position and role at work had come to a natural end, and it felt right to concentrate on home life for a bit. The day after I finished work was the first time I made an appointment with the health visitor to get our referral to the audiologist and the speech clinic. And from that moment sprung forth a new (unpaid!) role – Principal Carer and Unqualified Speech Support Worker... It worked for us as a family – it hasn't come without any set-backs, of course – for one, we are a salary down, but... it had to be, and I think our family has benefitted from many of the sacrifices we've had to make.

Make some time each week where everyone can be together, doing 'normal' things, where the speech disorder is not apparent nor given any thought. Try to make time to have fun, and forget about the verbal dyspraxia. Watch a film as a family, go bowling, make a den in the kitchen. Wind down as much as possible at the weekends, and if you can, try to make some 'me' time so that you can recharge your batteries. Easier said than done if you have children, but if you are feeling run down as a parent, that has an impact on how the family runs in many ways.

> A Parent's Perspective

Sometimes, family and friends can be a tricky thing.

In my experience, there are three different responses you may be likely to come across when you are telling those close to you that your child has been diagnosed with verbal dyspraxia. The first, and the most favourable, is the person who listens, sympathizes, and doesn't judge.

The second type of response may come from others whose reaction may be to try to make you feel better - which often means suggesting all manner of excuses - 'She *can* speak, she's just being lazy', or 'He's not speaking yet because he has an older sibling to do all the talking.' Some might also point out famous people who lived centuries ago that were late talkers. Sometimes these people have a friend of a friend who had a lisp and a tongue-tie when they were little, and they grew out of it by the age of eight. Not relevant, and not necessarily helpful, but I suppose they are just showing that they care.

The last type of response, and the one that used to frustrate me the most, is *denial*. A complete disregard and disbelief in the diagnosis - a condition that they may never have heard of - and the fact that there is nothing else wrong with the child and they just need to 'catch up'. It is very frustrating to have to explain that your child is not lazy, nor doing it on purpose, nor in some way 'intellectually challenged'.

In the case of the last response, you might want to lend them a copy of this book or another personal account such as *Anything but Silent: Our Family's Journey Through Childhood Apraxia of Speech* by Kathy and Kate Hennessy (Word Association Publishers, 2013) or point them in the direction of some relevant pages on the Internet such as those found on www.apraxia-kids.org.

Siblings

Depending on the age of any siblings or other children in the house, take time to explain it properly, in a way they will understand. Often children worry about things that as adults we wouldn't even think about. It can be difficult in a busy week, but do try as often as possible to make time to be with them on their own. Get them involved, give them helping jobs to do. Monty's brother likes to help him with his speech worksheets, and to read to him and play snap or other games that we have told him will help Monty.

Sometimes, siblings might be jealous of the attention given to their brother or sister. Ask them to be the note-taker at any family meetings for any outcomes that need 'recording', or to be responsible for filing the speech therapy worksheets. Giving them a job, and a purpose in all this mayhem, can work wonders.

They may feel worried about their brother or sister, and protective of them. I hadn't really thought about this, until Monty's teacher asked me if I could have a word with Monty's older brother, who was constantly inviting Monty to play with boys two years older than him in another playground at school, as he thought he needed to 'keep an eye on him!'

Conversely, there may be times when a sibling is worried about what their own friends think of their sibling – they may be embarrassed of their 'baby' speech, and their friends may make fun of them. If you work on being a close-knit family, and include them as much as possible, this should hopefully not pose too much of a problem.

I think it is important to explain why sometimes their sibling may be frustrated, but that it is not ok for their brother or sister to lash out at them, or somehow take it out on them, in case they find themselves bearing the brunt of any tantrums.

Make sure that you tell them how much you love them, that they are equally important, and how much of a help that you find them to be.

Grandparents

Grandparents may feel equally confused as to what their role might be in helping with your child with verbal dyspraxia. Give them some pointers on how to speak to the child, as they may feel uncomfortable about what to do, or worried that they will somehow offend. It may have been a long time since they had young children to look after, and with that may present a feeling that 'it'll just happen when the child is ready' or such-like. From the beginning, try to explain the condition as clearly as you can, along with the prognosis and length of time that it is perhaps likely to take in speech therapy. Explain how they can help, giving them some pointers of what to say to help correct speech errors, and importantly how to make sure they are not unwittingly giving negative feedback to the child.

Grandparents may want to help in other ways – they might offer to help pay for some private speech therapy, for instance, which you may find extremely helpful, or they may be willing to help you do some research.

Friends

We have been extremely fortunate to have some lovely friends who have been a good shoulder of support when things have been tough, and looking back I am glad that we involved those who cared about Monty from the beginning rather than hiding away and trying to deal with everything on our own. I think the above suggestions for grandparents also apply here, too, as those that care will only want to help you. If they don't, then perhaps they aren't the type of friends that you need right now, hey?

****

Chapter 8

Diet and Nutrition

In this section you might find some information on diet and nutrition that may come as something completely new to you – I have to say, it was a whole new world when I began to look into it, and to make some changes to the way in which I viewed Monty's diet . I must point out again that I am not a nutritionist, a doctor nor any other medical professional. I have always sort medical guidance when looking for alternative treatments, and it is important that you do the same, as what is right for one individual may not be so for another, so please view the following information about Monty's dietary and nutritional changes as a guide for undertaking your own research, and for contacting a relevant professional if it is something that you are interested in considering further.

> ➢ **Parents perspective**

At some point, I think you start to wonder if there is anything else you can possibly do to help your child. In my case, I started to wonder, *What's the missing link? What is it that I've missed?*

As you'll see throughout this chapter, there were many changes that we could make to Monty's diet that were receiving positive feedback from other parents. Once I started to implement the new diet at home, it was then necessary to think about the other places that Monty was eating. At nursery, they sent me to the kitchen to talk to the chef, who was very happy to put Monty on a gluten-free diet (there were several other children at the time following the same as us) and straight away he was put onto it.

Easy! Before Monty started at school, I went in to talk to the school office, and was told that I had to get permission from the County Council as they provide the food and I would need a medical note in order to do so.

At this point I was a little worried – I spoke to Monty's paediatrician and whilst she was happy for him to try a gluten-free diet, it wasn't a medical necessity (like a food allergy or intolerance that could be 'proved' or backed-up by test results.) She did, however, give me a letter that outlined why, as Monty's parents, we wanted to give it a go. On the day of the meeting with the Council, I was a little fidgety. What if they said no? Would I have to give him a packed lunch, and have him miss out on hot dinners in the winter? (My mother was a stickler for hot dinners in cold weather, and I seem to have inherited that gene!) As it turned out, I needn't have worried. The man we saw was very understanding, and after telling him about the research I had done about the positive effects other parents had found in their own children, he said that he was happy to put Monty on gluten-free meals, as he felt that the correct diet was very important for each individual child. I could have hugged him – very few meetings with other people involved in Monty's care had gone so well before this, and it felt great to not feel like I'd had to fight for it. Another reason to be prepared before any meeting about your child – doing your research and having your key aims, arguments and topics for discussion can really pay off.

Gluten
Gluten is a type of protein found in wheat and wheat-related products and grains, including rye and barley. It's a glue-like substance that binds things together and gives things a chewy texture, and helps bread to rise. Gluten is a hidden product in many

products, from make-up to some tomato ketchups, beers, and vinegars and many junk foods like crisps, ice-cream and chocolate. Gluten is well-known for cross-contamination in foods, which is often why some foods that do not contain gluten by nature (for example oats) can become contaminated in the production or factory process. In the UK, cereals must be labelled, but it is voluntary for companies to list gluten within other products.

Gluten gets a bad name because of the effect that it has on those suffering from coeliac disease, which can cause bloating, stomach discomfort, vomiting and diarrhoea amongst other symptoms. According to the charity Coeliac UK, 1 in 100 people are likely to have coeliac disease,[33] which is a lifelong autoimmune condition affecting the small intestine. In a nutshell, the body reacts badly to the gluten put into it, and the immune system starts to work against it. When a person is diagnosed with the condition via testing, the only solution is to follow a gluten-free diet for life. It is not a food allergy or intolerance.

Gluten sensitivity (non-coeliac) can occur in some people when eating gluten, although they do not have coeliac disease. It is generally agreed that it isn't clear how the immune system is involved, or if there is damage to the gut. There are lots of helpful leaflets, shopping guides and food lists that you can and can't eat on www.coeliac.org.uk.

Is there a link between gluten and verbal dyspraxia?
It would appear that there is some evidence, yes, and this is being strengthened with the more research being done. It seems that in some cases, children suffering with verbal dyspraxia may often find

---

[33] www.coeliac.org.uk/coeliac-disease (retrieved from website November 2014)

their symptoms are part of a wider-spread neurologic syndrome involving food allergies, possible gluten-sensitivity and nutritional malabsorption.

Malabsorption

One study in recent years noted increased speech in children with verbal dyspraxia (and some related conditions) when supplemented with controlled doses of vitamin E and polyunsaturated fatty acids. The report (see footnote) states that, 'Vitamin E deficiency causes symptoms that overlap those of verbal apraxia. Polyunsaturated fatty acids in the cell membrane are vulnerable to lipid peroxidation and early destruction if vitamin E is not readily available, potentially leading to neurological sequelae. Inflammation of the gastrointestinal (GI) tract and malabsorption of nutrients such as vitamin E and carnitine may contribute to neurological abnormalities.[34]

I'm fascinated by the idea that there could be a connection between the gut and brain. A good article to read is by C R Morris and M C Agin, *Syndrome Of Allergy, Apraxia, And Malabsorption: Characterization Of A Neurodevelopmental Phenotype That Responds To Omega 3 And Vitamin E Supplementation*, which can be found by putting the title into a search engine on the internet.

---

[34] http://www.ncbi.nlm.nih.gov/pubmed/19623831 - C R Morris and M C Agin - Syndrome of allergy, apraxia, and malabsorption: characterization of a neurodevelopmental phenotype that responds to omega 3 and vitamin E supplementation. (Featured in Alternative Therapies, July/August 2009

Casein

Casein is the main protein found in milk and cheese products, and a contributor to many milk and whey allergies. There is much anecdotal evidence from other parents that following both a gluten-free and casein-free diet can help greatly in the treatment of verbal dyspraxia. Personally, I always thought that we would need to move on from just cutting out the gluten but for us that was been all we need for now to get the ball rolling. For some reason, even though Monty doesn't drink much milk or eat much cheese, this seemed so much harder to cut out than the gluten. But I reserve the right to look at this again in the future (just in case!).

Brain food

Coeliac Matters, a website from the USA, states that, 'anecdotally the speech of children with verbal apraxia will often improve dramatically when they take high-quality fish oil.[35] I have to say, within a month of putting Monty onto a good quality fish oil supplement, with Omega 3 and Omega 6, we noticed a difference in the clarity of his speech.

Fatty acid testing can identify which nutritional deficiencies your child may be suffering from in terms of omega 3 and omega 6, as well as other essential fats. There are testing kits available that you can purchase to do this.

Always consult with your child's doctor and a qualified nutritionist before embarking on any changes to your child's diet, or before introducing any supplements.

---

[35] Www.coeliacmatters.com, *Apraxia appears to be linked to food allergies, gluten sensitivity and nutrient malabsorption* (retrieved from website in December 2014)

Nutritional Therapy

'Nutritional therapy is a functional medicine approach based on current scientific research that promotes optimal health and peak performance. Registered Nutritional Therapists use a wide range of tools to assess and identify potential nutritional imbalances and understand how these may be contributing to an individual's symptoms and health concerns. This approach enables the development of a bespoke programme addressing an individual's unique needs. Practitioner's toolkits include reviewing signs and symptoms, dietary intake and functional tests. Testing also helps to develop suitable supplement programmes if necessary.'

Written by Katharine Tate, Nutritionist, The Food Teacher

The Food Teacher Clinic provides access to Registered Nutritional Therapists with experience of a range of neurodevelopmental conditions including apraxia. Face-to-face or Skype consultations can be provided depending on location. Information can be found at www.thefoodteacher.co.uk
Other registered Nutritional Therapists can be found at:

- British Association for Applied Nutrition and Nutritional Therapy (BANT) - http://bant.org.uk

- Nutritionist Resource (All nutritionists are members of a recognised professional body) - http://www.nutritionist-resource.org.uk/

- Complementary and Natural Healthcare Council (CNHC) - http://www.cnhc.org.uk

Background to introducing a new diet

Katharine Tate was the nutritionist that I approached to help with Monty's diet. As well as being a good friend, she has an excellent
144

understanding of the do's and don'ts for feeding the brain the correct food. She has kindly contributed the following to give an experts view on the importance of putting the correct nutrients into a child's diet, especially when there is a neurological condition, and the impact of food on brain development. Katharine writes:

'You are what you eat is time and time again used to reference the importance of the foods we consume and whilst we are aware of the value of our diet to our overall health it is easy to forget how vast its contribution is in relation to the overall optimum functioning of our bodies, especially our brains. If key nutrients are deficient from our diets - or even at birth - our body will utilise the resources it has but eventually it will reach a tipping point where it can no longer maintain balance, which may ultimately emanate in disorder and disease.

Our brain takes priority above all other organs and is the biggest fuel source demander in our bodies utilising 20% of our oxygen and calorie intake.[36] Nutrients and growth factors not only regulate brain development during foetal and early postnatal life, but also help to sustain efficiency of the brain throughout life.[37] Rapidly developing brains are more vulnerable to nutrient insufficiency or overabundance so nutrient status and timing is

---

[36] Raichle M E, Gusnard D A (2002) Appraising the brain's energy budget. *Proceedings of the National Academy of Sciences*, *99*: 10237-10239. Also, Magistretti P J, Allaman I (2013) Brain energy metabolism. In: *Neuroscience in the 21st Century.* Springer New York, p 1591-1620.

[37] Georgieff M K (2007) Nutrition and the developing brain: nutrient priorities and measurement. *The American journal of clinical nutrition*, *85*: 614S-620S.

essential and the remarkable plasticity of a young child's brain may provide a window of opportunity to repair nutrient depletion. Not only do nutrients develop the structure of the brain they also provide cofactors for the enzymes in the brain that convert foods we eat into the body's required building blocks.

Basic brain structure is laid down by 50% genetics and 50% environment (epigenetics). Whilst our inherited genetic behaviour is fixed our control over environmental factors is huge when we consider diet, hydration, learning opportunities, exercise, control of toxin exposure and stress.[38]

The human brain starts developing around one month after conception and continues to develop until early adulthood. During the last trimester to age two the brain undergoes a significant 'brain growth spurt', which initially prepares the baby for survival, including breathing and suckling and then for sensorimotor cognitive growth.

Certain nutrients have greater effect on brain development than others and an understanding of these factors can raise an awareness of our child's nutrient exposure, which may help to address any potential imbalances and provide some restorative benefits. The health of our brain is also interrelated to all other systems in our body and significant research has focused on the gut-brain axis and the health of our digestive system, which have been

---

[38] Shannon S M (2013) Parenting the Whole Child: A Holistic Child Psychiatrist Offers Practical Wisdom on Behavior, Brain Health, Nutrition, Exercise, Family Life, Peer Relationships, School Life, Trauma, Medication, and More. W. W Norton & Company Inc., New York, p31.

linked to our behaviour and neurodevelopmental disorders.[39] Therefore, considering what we do and don't eat is important for our brain structure and most significant for children with potential neurodevelopmental imbalances such as apraxia.'

Katharine continues,

'I started to work with Sam a few years ago when signs suggested Monty's speech was not developing in-line with his peers. Initial consultations focused on Sam's diet, pregnancy and labour which helped us to build a picture of his health status and potential imbalances. We carried out some functional tests to assess his overall nutrient status and his fatty acid profile and then intervened with dietary advice and supplementation. This alongside all the other interventions Sam has worked so hard to implement has had a huge impact on his development and each time we meet it is fantastic to hear about the progress he is making day by day.'

Here is a table that Katharine developed for Monty, to enable me to ensure that he was eating the right types of food for him.

See overleaf.

---

[39] Stilling R M, Dinan T G, Cryan J F (2014) Microbial genes, brain & behaviour–epigenetic regulation of the gut–brain axis. *Genes, Brain and Behavior*, 13: 69-86

Key Brain Foods[40]
(A balance of nutrients is essential as they work synergistically in the body to support optimal health)

Macronutrients

Nutrient	Function	Rich Food Sources
Protein	Provide the building blocks for our bodies. Needed for growth and repair of body tissues, brain chemical messengers, hormones and enzymes.	Meat Dairy Legumes – beans, chickpeas Wholegrains Nuts and seeds
Fats (60% of dry weight of brain is fat)	A good balance of polyunsaturated, monosaturated and saturated is needed for membrane structure, brain and nerve function, mood, energy and	Meat (grass-fed) Fish Dairy Foods Coconut Oil Avocados Nuts and seeds Olive oil Green Leafy

[40] Table references:

Murray M, Pizzorno J, Pizzorno L (2005) *The encyclopaedia of healing foods.* London, Piatkus.
Georgieff M K (2007) Nutrition and the developing brain: nutrient priorities and measurement. *The American journal of clinical nutrition, 85*: 614S-620S.

	metabolism. Helps us to absorb fat soluble vitamins A, D E and K.	Vegetables
Essential Fatty Acids (25% is brain is DHA-Docosahexaenoic acid – Omega-3)	Important structural and functional role in the brain. Reduces inflammation, supports metabolism and reduces oxidative stress. Body inefficient at synthesizing DHA, reliant on diet.	Oily fish – Salmon, tuna, mackerel Flaxseed Pumpkin seeds Walnuts
Carbohydrates	Provides glucose and fuel for the brain providing neurons with power. Healthier choice is to choose complex carbohydrates rather than white, processed grains.	Wholegrains – rice, pasta, bread Oats Potatoes Legumes Cereal
Micronutrients		

Nutrient	**Function**	**Rich Food Sources**
Iron	Needed to modulate cerebral development, supply	Clams

	of oxygen to the brain and increasing brain energy production. Cognitive performance and low iron levels and autism under research. Vitamin C enhances absorption.	Molasses Nuts and seeds Liver Egg yolks Red Meat (grass-fed) Legumes Lentils
Zinc	Abundant in the brain contributing to structure and function. Supports healthy immunity, growth, repair, circulation, eyes, skin, joints, metabolism and hormones. Some studies have shown supplementation can impact on cognition.	Oysters Ginger Red meat (grass-fed) Nuts and seeds Legumes
B Vitamins	B vitamins work together to maintain the health of our nervous system and brain. Deficiencies are linked to neurological disease.	Yeast extract (marmite) Liver Fish – Tuna Meat Nuts and seeds Wholegrains Avocado

Vitamin B12 – Cobalamin	Used for cell formation including red blood cells, therefore important for healthy nervous system. (Plants do not contain bioactive forms – imp. for vegans to supplement/fortified foods, e.g. marmite)	Liver Shellfish Oily fish Eggs Meat Dairy
Choline	Needed for brain chemical messengers and brain cell structure.	Eggs Prawns Chicken
Magnesium	Structure and metabolic role important for brain health. Also needed for tissue repair and energy production.	Kelp Seaweed Nuts and seeds Spinach Apricots Dates Avocado
Copper	Needed for iron absorption, red blood cells, motor function, coordination and balance.	Nuts and seeds Butter Legumes

Selenium	Antioxidant important for thyroid health and body repair.	Oats Tuna Garlic Eggs
Vitamin A	Antioxidant, which quenches damaging free radicals.	Liver Carrots Apricots Dark green leafy vegetables Fish
Vitamin D	Protects the brain neurons and modulates the transport of glucose. Area of on-going research.	Oily fish Seeds Dairy Mushrooms
Phytonutrients – Plant chemicals – e.g. quercitin, flavonols	As the brain has such a high metabolic load it is susceptible to oxidative damage which phytonutrients help to quench acting as antioxidants.	Rainbow of fruit and vegetables Berries Grapes Beans Onions Plums Cranberries

In contrast, here are the foods that it was suggested we try to limit or avoid:

Brain 'Anti-nutrients'
(These 'anti-nutrients' may have damaging effects on brain development, though the extent of their effect is dependent on individual biochemistry.)

Anti-nutrients/Toxin

Nutrient/Toxin	Potential Effect	Sources
Artificial Sweeteners	Research suggests they can compromise the blood brain barrier increasing permeability, increasing oxidative stress load and stimulating neurodegeneration.[41]	Asparatme, saccharin, acesulfame-K, sucralose, neotame – often found in diet/low-fat drinks and foods
Gluten	Gluten has been shown to trigger an immune response in some individuals increasing inflammation and directly harming the	Foods containing flour (pasta, bread, cakes, biscuits), couscous, cereal, crackers, beer, oats (can be cross contaminated), gravy,

[41] Humphries P, Pretorius E, Naude H (2007) Direct and indirect cellular effects of aspartame on the brain. *European journal of clinical nutrition*, 62: 451-462.

	brain and nervous system.[42]	dressings, sauces
Trans fats	Trans fats compete with DHA in the brain affecting cell fluidity and electrical activity. This can affect nervous system communication, increase stress levels and prepare the brain for early degeneration.[43]	Foods that contain hydrogenated or partially hydrogenated vegetable fats to increase shelf life of foods – deep fried foods, some take away meals, some baked foods such as biscuits, pies, pastries, cakes and biscuits
Other		
Toxin Exposure (chemicals, toxins and pollutants)	Chemical and heavy metals accumulate in the body and can affect neurotransmitter	Perfumes, toiletries (shower gels, shampoos, lotions), cleaning products, pollutants in the

[42] Hadjivassiliou M, Sanders D S, Grünewald R A. Woodroofe N, Boscolo S, Aeschlimann D (2010) Gluten sensitivity: from gut to brain. *The Lancet Neurology*, 9: 318-330.

[43] Bowman G L, Silbert L C, Howieson D, Dodge H H, Traber M G, Frei B, Quinn J F (2012) Nutrient biomarker patterns, cognitive function, and MRI measures of brain aging. *Neurology*, 78:241-249

	function. Increased toxic effects can be linked to poor liver function, increased blood brain barrier permeability and inflammation.[44]	environment and on our food etc.
Lack of exercise	Brain needs oxygen for cells to complete basic functions. If sedentary cells can be deprived and may not receive enough for optimal development. Exercise benefits include increased brain plasticity.[45]	-
Stress	Linked to predisposition to various mental	-

[44] Weiss B, Landrigan P J (2000) The developing brain and the environment: an introduction. *Environmental health perspectives*, 108: 373.

[45] Cotman C W, Berchtold N C, Christie L A (2007). Exercise builds brain health: key roles of growth factor cascades and inflammation. *Trends in neurosciences*, 30: 464-472.

[46] Wright L, Perrot T (2012) Stress and the Developing Brain. In: *Colloquium Series on The Developing Brain* (Vol. 3, No. 3, pp. 1-76). Morgan & Claypool Life Sciences.

	illnesses such as depression and anxiety. Can increase inflammation, impair blood glucose levels and increase blood brain barrier permeability. [46]	
Dehydration	Brain shrinkage can occur if not adequately hydrated which can impact on brain and cognitive function.[47]	Water

Daily food ideas that Katharine suggested we try to include
Breakfast:
- Eggs
- Salmon
- Fruit and yoghurt
- Porridge
- Smoothies (choose low sugar fruits such as berries, include avocados, dark green leafy vegetables)

Lunch:
- Fish

---

[47] Popkin B M, D'Anci K E, Rosenberg I H (2010). Water, hydration, and health. *Nutrition reviews*, 68: 439-458

- Meat (choose grass-fed for higher omega-3's)
- Vegetables
- Wholegrains (brown rice, wholewheat pasta)

Dinner:
- Fish
- Meat (choose grass-fed for higher omega-3's)
- Legumes
- Lentils
- Vegetables
- Wholegrains (brown rice, wholewheat pasta)

Snacks:
- Nuts/seeds
- Fruit/vegetables
- Yoghurt
- Dips (guacamole, hummus)
- Smoothies

So ultimately, what did we decide to do for Monty?

Katharine undertook a full consultation for Monty, starting with our extended family history, my pregnancy, labour and birth, all the way through to Monty's early months of life, to the present day. She did an assessment of Monty's stools, which were very hard and difficult to pass, and we undertook functional tests which are described below.

<u>A note on Functional Tests</u>

With the help of a nutritional therapist appropriate functional laboratory tests can be identified and performed. Such tests can be invaluable in identifying potential causes to health imbalances and may facilitate faster steps towards optimum health. Typical tests involve a breath, blood, saliva, urine or stool sample and can often be carried out at home.

Some of the tests that may be considered for neurodevelopmental disorders include:

- **Nutritional and Toxin Status Assessment**

An imbalance of nutrients and high levels of toxins such as heavy metals have been implicated in health conditions including depression and behavioural disorders. The test analyses a urine sample looking for specific markers which includes measures for vitamin and mineral status, protein adequacy, cellular energy production, neurotransmitter processing, liver function and gut bacteria balance.

- **Fatty Acids Profile**

This test measures fatty acid profile using a blood sample, which can be a fingertip home testing kit. The tests give an indicator of omega-3 levels, the ratio of omega-6/3 and levels of trans fats. Such information is a good indicator of inflammation in the body and as 25% of the brain is Docosahexaenoic acid (DHA) an awareness of levels can support a more targeted supplementation programme.

- **Gastrointestinal Tests**

Evaluating intestinal health may help to improve overall health specifically in relation to the brain and the gut-brain axis. Areas which testing may support include potential malabsorption of nutrients, constipation, irritable bowel, control of fungal and parasitic infections.

- **Immunology Tests**

Food and environmental allergens have been linked to a whole host of conditions that can be far reaching in the body. Different antibody profiles can be performed to identify allergic reactions and intolerances including the most common allergens such as milk, egg, wheat, soy, fish and shellfish.

(The laboratories that I know of that do these types of tests include: Genova Diagnostics, Biolab, HQT Diagnostics and Regenerus Laboratories). In Monty's case, we decided on the following:

1) We had him tested for nutritional deficiencies:

- Fatty Acid analysis (home testing kit with a pin-prick test, to look at levels of essential fatty acids Omega-6 and Omega-3 and trans fats levels) -we used the HGT diagnostics test (www.hqt-diagnostics.com) which was sent away, and the results received in two weeks. Interestingly, the Fatty Acids test was undertaken after being gluten-free for 9 months whilst taking the fish oils and other supplements, and his levels came back really good!

- Amino acid urine test to get a picture of the nutritional deficiencies, toxins, digestive function, metabolic analysis. I used the Genova Diagnostics laboratory, which involved taking a urine sample which was then frozen and sent away for testing. From this a detailed plan of the necessary supplements was devised by Katharine.

2) Blood tests were undertaken to establish his iron levels

3) 'The Sweetcorn Test' - to see how fast or slow the body's digestive system is working. I gave Monty a normal portion of sweetcorn with his dinner, and had to check his stools to see the first signs of sweetcorn emerging (the things we do for our

children!)Sweetcorn does not dissolve properly and therefore is easy to see when going to the toilet. It took three times the normal length of time for the sweetcorn to be visible, and it was evident that Monty needed some help to move things along, as it were.

Individual strategy

Following on from the above, we implemented the following. **Please note - this was a nutritional plan put in place for Monty as an individual, and I list it here for the purpose of showing an example of the type of strategy that may be put in place should you choose to follow the same type of testing.**

Monty was put on an initial 3 month strategy, which looked at the following:

- Removing potential gut irritants by eliminating gluten
- increasing bulk in the stool to help Monty 'go'
- Improve 'transit time' when Monty 'goes' by helping the gut wall to be lubricated
- Increase digestive enzyme production
- Help liver detoxification
- Increasing the 'brain foods' into Monty's diet
- Supporting identified nutritional deficiencies found in the test results, which included:

The following were introduced:

1) Fish oil - we have used a brand called Eskimo 'Brainsharp', to supplement his omega fatty acids for brain development and overall health.

2) Magnesium spray to replace his body's low magnesium level.

3) Probiotics to heal the digestive system and potential 'leaky gut.' It appears that there is a link between the gut leaking contents of the stomach into the bloodstream, which leads to toxins travelling to places in the body that they shouldn't be. The journal on Allergy, Apraxia and Malabsorption previously mentioned states that 'the impact of abnormal gut flora and inflammation on the gastrointestinal (GI) tract may contribute to damage of the mucosal lining that leads to increased permeability or a "leaky gut, which allows the abnormal passage of molecules from the GI tract into the bloodstream, triggers the development of multiple food allergies, and feeds the cycle of inflammation.[48]

4) Introducing a general vitamin supplement which suited the deficiencies found in the amino acid test.

What happened?
Quite frankly, we were amazed at the positive effect the changes to Monty's diet seemed to make. His nursery saw an improvement in his concentration and clarity of sounds within a week of going gluten-free. We need more research into the effect on diet and nutrition in cases of verbal dyspraxia, and then hopefully the medical world will start to sit up and listen, as there are many practitioners and parents of children with verbal dyspraxia (and other conditions) who are convinced of the benefits of making these types of changes.

---

[48] http://www.ncbi.nlm.nih.gov/pubmed/19623831 - C R Morris and M C Agin - Syndrome of allergy, apraxia, and malabsorption: characterization of a neurodevelopmental phenotype that responds to omega 3 and vitamin E supplementation. (Alternative Therapies, July/August 2009)

Books to read

I like the recipes and food and diet information given in the Patrick Holford books. Have a look at *Smart Food for Smart Kids* (Patrick Holford, Piatkus, 2007) and *Optimum Nutrition for your Child's Mind* (Patrick Holford, Piatkus, 2005).

Another good one to have a look at is *Autism: Exploring the Benefits of a Gluten- and Casein-Free Diet* (Paul Whitely, Mark Earnden, Elouise Robinson, Routledge, 2014). Although the book is primarily about the effects of an alternative diet on the presentation and characteristics of autism, it gives a good insight into the science and benefits of going gluten and casein-free. Verbal dyspraxia is often called a 'cousin' of autism, ADHD and Asperger's due to the similarities in the neurological remit, and the fact than in many cases, verbal dyspraxia can run hand-in-hand with any of these conditions. There are also some good recipe ideas in the book to get you going.

****

Chapter 9

Looking to the Future

➢ A parent's perspective

At the time of writing, Monty is four years and three months old. He has been in the Reception class at school for around eight weeks, and over the last four weeks, we have seen some amazing progress, which has astounded us and both his speech and language therapists. Monty can now say a variety of short sentences, and has now realised 'd', 't', 'b', 'c' and 'p' which he has worked on for so long. To put it into context, we have spent the last fourteen months learning to blow, working on the sounds 's' and 'sh', and achieving three vowel sounds. And that was mostly it, in terms of output for the majority of that period of time. Until now.

Monty can now say his own name, and his brother's name. He can ask for more food, say that he is dizzy when he spins round and round, and tell me why he is cross/happy/sad. He can tell me some of the names of the children he plays with, and can say the surname of his teacher. He even has a line to say in the school Christmas play, which his teacher said he volunteered for, even though they gave him the choice of taking a silent role... Somehow, from the depths of nowhere it seems, we have had a breakthrough.

I had the shock of my life, just a few days ago, when we were all watching a Disney movie as a family. I happened to mention that the birds in the jungle - lovely bright little birds that were nesting high up in the trees - were really pretty. From the corner of the sofa a little voice piped up. 'Not birds, Mummy - parrots. They *parrots*.' It was Monty, and all of us looked down to

163

the end of the sofa in surprise - and what a lovely surprise it was. Monty, in his own little way, seems to give a little smile when he speaks his words these days, as if he knows that what he's doing is a major triumph; the culmination of months and months of hard work, and - well, that he knows it's just a little bit special for all of us to hear him. When I set out to write this book, I had no idea how the final chapter would go, and whether or not I would have any changes to write about in terms of his current level of progress.

It's funny, because sometimes it's the little things that can really stop me in my tracks. I seemed to have become quite hardened in my approach to Monty's verbal dyspraxia - it became a project, a massive mountain to overcome that required dogged determination, step-by-step analysis, and time management skills worthy of the most diligent personal assistant. Perhaps this approach made it easier to deal with - almost as if I could become detached from the situation, and in doing so could get on with the job a little bit easier. It is only when I see something on the TV, perhaps a *Children in Need* clip where a child is struggling to speak, or an advert, or a programme like *Educating Yorkshire*, which showed a teenager overcoming a stammer to finally talk in front of his peers, that the enormity of Monty's communication disorder really seems to hit home. I think it's a bit like referred pain, when the feeling is only apparent and perceived via another source, which serves as a reminder of my usually hidden feelings that are tucked well away from the surface. In a way, it's been a good coping mechanism as a parent, although not necessarily a conscious decision.

We know that we are not out of the woods yet, by any means. The past has taught me that there will be set-backs along the way - we've seen regression, whereby Monty (seemingly overnight) lost the handful of words that he had, for several weeks;

and we've had a prolonged period of selective mutism whereby Monty refused to speak in clinic, becoming very suspicious of anyone who remotely looked like a speech therapist (carrying a clipboard, a box of animals, or a desk full of stacking bricks...) We've also had periods of frustration so bad that I have dreaded us leaving the house in the morning. Every two steps forward seem to carry a promise of one step back. Sometimes when we finish working on a certain sound, and we leave it alone for a short time, we seem to need to revisit it, and reinforce it again, rather than just being able to tick it off the list as completed.

It seems inevitable at the moment that Monty is perhaps moving towards having an expressive language disorder. I can tell from his speech that as the words are coming, there is a difficulty in putting them in the right order, especially if his sentence is more than three or four words long. Just as you think you are getting somewhere, along comes something else to nip at your heels! At the moment, I can only explain it by saying that sometimes Monty talks in the same sentence structure as Yoda from *Star Wars* – he might say something like 'Home I go now', or 'Doggy here come now in.' Our next meeting with the school, Monty's speech and language therapists and u as parents, is set for next month, and we will be reviewing his targets and action plan and therapy sessions to ensure that everyone involved is concentrating on sentence structure and formation now, as things are now moving in a different direction. As the condition morphs and changes, so must the approach to treat it.

I worry about the future, and whether this sustained level of progress will continue. I worry about whether Monty will progress from infant school to the juniors, happy in the knowledge that he is making enough progress to keep up with his peers. I worry that his verbal dyspraxia will develop into another associated form of speech disorder, and that his expressive language delay will become more apparent as he works on his literacy, spelling and reading, and as his sentences that he can say start to get longer. I worry that the four and five years olds, who are so helpful, accommodating and kind to Monty at the moment, will start to see that he is different in some ways to them, and that he will suffer because of other people's perceptions of him. Above all, I worry about whether he will be happy, and confident, and able to achieve all of the dreams he will have in the future.

Knowing last night that I was going to write this chapter today, I tried to think of one example in the evening that would signify that we had somehow 'won', something that would be my 'cherry on the cake' moment, whereby I would know that we were really kicking Monty's verbal dyspraxia into touch. And it came to me whilst I was getting both my sons ready for bed. I was upstairs, sorting out the washing and running a bath, whilst simultaneously searching for toothbrushes and shouting to the boys to join me in the bathroom. I heard my eldest son shout a long, protracted reason as to why it wasn't convenient for him to come up for a bath, and why he had a handful of pressing things to do in the playroom ('Nice try!' was my answer, directly followed by 'Get upstairs now!'). Monty, on the other hand, said a quiet 'Ok, mummy', and made his way up the stairs, ready to do what was asked, because sometimes I think it seems that it is easier for him to do what is asked of him rather than find the words to talk about it, even if, deep-down, he'd really rather not.

And that was when it hit me – the day that I hear a protesting voice from another room in the house, with a reasoned argument as to why they as an individual should not have to have a bath/take the dog out/do their homework, and I don't know *which* son it has come from, then that day will be my 'eureka' moment.

My two sons appear to have voices that are quite similar in tone and pitch, and when the words and sentences and conversations also start to come out the same, well – it won't get much better than that.

It might not seem like much but, sometimes, it's the small things that pack the biggest punch.

****

Chapter 10

Further Reading and Information

Groups, Organisations and Professional Bodies

- Speech Therapists - Royal College of Speech and Language Therapists - www.rcslt.org
- The Nuffield Centre - Information on the Nuffield Centre based from the Royal National Throat, Nose and Ear Hospital in London. The NDP3 programme was developed as a programme for Speech and Language Therapists for managing verbal dyspraxia. It consists of therapy cards and worksheets, alongside the Speech Builder computer programme.
- Dyspraxia Foundation www.dyspraxiafoundation.org.uk - Mostly focussing on full body dyspraxia but has one or two mentions on speech and language. In the 'downloads' section, have a look under 'Developmental Verbal Dyspraxia' where you can read Pam William's information sheet. Pam is a Principal Speech and Language Therapist at the Nuffield Hearing and Speech Centre. The sheet includes some oromotor exercises to be getting on with while you are waiting to see a Speech and Language Therapist
- Apraxia Kids (CASANA) www.apraxia-kids.org - Probably the most useful website I've ever come across. CASANA is the Childhood Apraxia of Speech Association of North America. An absolute wealth of information! Really interesting to see the differences in the information available here in the UK

and in the USA. Check out the 'Family Start Guide' which is a really comprehensive beginner's guide to verbal dyspraxia (or Childhood Apraxia of Speech as it is known there.) Loads of downloads and brochures which are really helpful for handing out to family members and teacher etc. to explain the condition. The download, *'If I Could Only Tell You, I Would Say'* which aims to get across the likely views of a child with verbal dyspraxia always makes me cry...

- www.afasic.org.uk
- Nutritional Therapists - British Association for Applied Nutrition and Nutritional Therapy (BANT), Complementary and Natural Healthcare Council (CNHC)
- The Makaton Charity - www.makaton.org.
- I CAN (The Children's Communication Charity) – www.ican.org.uk

Useful Books

- *Speaking of Apraxia – A Parent's Guide to Childhood Apraxia of Speech* – by Leslie A. Lindsay (Woodbine House, 2012). A really good read. I especially liked the section on alternative/complementary practices and diets.
- *Anything but Silent* – by Kathy and Kate Hennessy (Word Association Publishers, 2013.) Written by a mother and a now teenage daughter, this is a heart-warming (and somewhat heart-breaking) account of one family's journey with apraxia. Really nice to read about it from a child's perspective.
- *Mouth and Tongue Let's Have Some Fun!* – Karina Hopper (Jessica Kingsley Publishers, 2010). A short book on mouth and tongue exercises. Quite similar to the Mr Tongue story.

- *The 50 Best Games for Speech and Language Development* – Maria Monschein (Hinton House, 2008.) Some good ideas here for games to play at home, encouraging mouth movements and also fine motor skills.
- *The Late Talker: What to do if Your Child isn't Talking Yet* – Marilyn Agin, Lisa F Geng, Malcolm Nicholl (St Martin's Griffin, 2004)
- *A Parent's Guide to Speech and Language Problems* – Debbie Feit (Mc-Craw-Hill, 2007
- *Childhood Speech, Language and Listening Problems – What every parent should know* – Patricia McAleer Hamaguchi (Jossey Bass, 3rd ed, 2010)
- *How to Identify and Support Children with Speech and Language Difficulties* – Jane Speake (LDA, 2003)
- *Teach Me How to Say It Right: Helping Your Child with Articulation Problems* - Dorothy P. Dougherty (New Harbinger, 2005)
- *The Mouth with a Mind of Its Own* – Patricia L. Mervine (Speaking of Speech.com, 2014) .A nice story for kids about a little boy starting school and his troubles with communicating and the misunderstandings that ensue with his new teacher and classmates.
- *My Brother is Very Special* – Amy Glorioso May (Trafford Publishing, 2004). I had to order this from America (the postage cost more than the book!). My other son took this into school for 'Show and Tell' to read to his classmates about his brother's condition. Quite short and therefore good for short attention spans!

Websites and Blogs

- My own blog, www.waiting-for-a-voice.com

- www.Jakes-journey-apraxia.com

- www.mommyspeechtherapy.com

- www.singinghands.co.uk - developed by two mum's of children with additional needs, they do baby signing classes and have developed a range of CDs and DVDs to enable children to sing and sign. I love the Christmas DVD.

Speech therapy aids

- Common sense media - 'Power up!' - Guide to the best apps for learning difficulties and special educational needs. https://www.commonsensemedia.org/guide/special-needs.

- Articulation Station app by Little Bee Speech

- My Choice Pad app - shows the Makaton symbol, a demonstration of how to reproduce the Makaton sign, and then an audio of the word. You can build sentences from the words so this can be a useful ...

Learning whilst playing

- Toy phones to speak into that play back what you said
- Talking Tunes CD (you ca find this on Amazon)

- What's Up? Game – you have to describe what picture is on someone else's headband
- Mr Tumble books, magazines, DVDs and CDs - *Something Special*.
- Sookie and Finn books and DVDs (you can find these on Amazon)

****

Index